100 Questions & Answers About Schizophrenia: Painful Minds

Second Edition

Lynn E. DeLisi, MD
Visiting Professor of Psychiatry
Harvard Medical School
Boston, Massachusetts
VA Boston Healthcare System
Brockton, Massachusetts

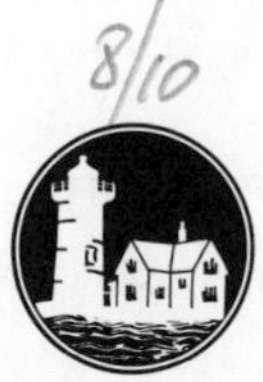

JONES AND BARTLETT PUBLISHERS
Sudbury, Massachusetts
BOSTON TORONTO LONDON SINGAPORE

World Headquarters
Jones and Bartlett Publishers
40 Tall Pine Drive
Sudbury, MA 01776
978-443-5000
info@jbpub.com
www.jbpub.com

Jones and Bartlett Publishers Canada
6339 Ormindale Way
Mississauga, Ontario L5V 1J2
Canada

Jones and Bartlett Publishers International
Barb House, Barb Mews
London W6 7PA
United Kingdom

Jones and Bartlett's books and products are available through most bookstores and online booksellers. To contact Jones and Bartlett Publishers directly, call 800-832-0034, fax 978-443-8000, or visit our website, www.jbpub.com.

Substantial discounts on bulk quantities of Jones and Bartlett's publications are available to corporations, professional associations, and other qualified organizations. For details and specific discount information, contact the special sales department at Jones and Bartlett via the above contact information or send an email to specialsales@jbpub.com.

Production Credits
Publisher: Christopher Davis
Editorial Assistant: Sara Cameron
Associate Production Editor: Sarah Bayle
Senior Marketing Manager: Barb Bartoszek
Manufacturing and Inventory Control Supervisor: Amy Bacus
Composition: Glyph International
Cover Design: Colleen Lamy
Cover Images: Top, © LiquidLibrary; bottom left, © Photos.com; bottom right, © Dreamstime Agency/Dreamstime.com
Printing and Binding: Malloy, Inc.
Cover Printing: Malloy, Inc.

Library of Congress Cataloging-in-Publication Data
DeLisi, Lynn E.
100 questions & answers about schizophrenia : painful minds / Lynn E. DeLisi.
p. cm. — (100 questions & answers)
Includes bibliographical references and index.
ISBN 978-0-7637-7657-2 (alk. paper)
1. Schizophrenia—Popular works. 2. Schizophrenia—Miscellanea. I. Title. II. Title: 100 questions and answers about schizophrenia. III. Title: One hundred questions & answers about schizophrenia.
RC514.D45 2010
616.89'8—dc22

2009038887

6048

Printed in the United States of America
13 12 11 10 09 10 9 8 7 6 5 4 3 2 1

Dedication

This volume is dedicated to all families worldwide who suffer because they have one or more relatives with schizophrenia, to those individuals whose lives have been destroyed by this illness, and to those professionals who have devoted their lives to the service of patients with serious mental illness.

Contents

A Sister's Perspective

This book is dedicated to the memory of many remarkable individuals, such as Scott David Shannon, a man of incredible courage, compassion, and intelligence. Growing up as his twin sister, I knew him well. Some of my first memories are of laughing with him while our young mom pushed us in a double stroller down the slightly sloping and bumpy village sidewalk of Shirley Street in Shortsville, New York. Scott and I held hands on our first day of kindergarten, were read to in our pajamas on either side of Mom while in bed, ran with other kids in the "pickle"-shaped park in the middle of our street during the afternoons, and often played Monopoly and other board games inside on rainy days. We had an easy middle-class life despite our father living separately in Maryland and only rarely calling, visiting, or providing any type of support. Scott and I had a stable and loving home, with our mother, Carol Ann, and grandfather, Elger, both working full time, and with our stay-at-home grandmother, Alice, doing the cooking and cleaning. I remember when our grandmother was making a yummy cake for dinner, she would offer Scott and me each one of the electronic mixing whisks to lick when we got home from school. Grandma Alice made sure we went to Sunday school and church. Our family life was not exactly tranquil, however, often with heated conversations over political and social issues argued over the dinner table or in the family living room.

In elementary school, Scott and I both found that good grades came to us easily, although like most children, we had to be told to do our homework. We both looked forward to summertime, with swimming in the neighbor's pools, the days at the Roseland amusement park, week-long vacations at the 4-H camp in Bristol Hills, and trips to the cabin on Blue Mountain Lake in the Adirondacks with our grandparents. In the mountains, Scott would go boating and fishing with Grandpa, and I would pick black-eyed Susan flowers and drink hot tea with Grandma. Once, Scott and I raced up Blue Mountain for about an hour and Scott emerged victorious, arriving at the summit first. We stayed on top of the mountain just long enough to see the view with the expanse of evergreen trees and shimmering lake below, but we could not wait to race back down, and I arrived at the bottom ahead of Scott!

We were generally in competition with each other in academics, as well. For example, in high school we both worked toward the best grade in algebra, which our grandfather forewarned us would be a "tough" subject. That year Scott was only 2 points behind my score of 100 on the state-wide Regents Exam in algebra, and a year later, I was 2 points behind his score of 98 in geometry. We both loved math and found the academic aspects of high school a lot less challenging than the social aspects. We were both physically small and not very athletic, and consequently we were often the last chosen for athletic teams, which did not help our self-esteem. I remember feeling awkward at my first teenage party, not knowing where to stand or who to talk to and being glad when it was over. When I was about 15 or 16, some neighborhood boys started hanging around my house and my best friend's house. I remember that my brother would stand on the front porch yelling at those boys to get off the lawn and I thought, "Why is he acting that way?"

My whole family (Grandpa, Grandma, and Mom) all smoked cigarettes, and so it was no surprise that Scott and I both tried cigarettes when we were teens. Scott got hooked on smoking at around 16 years of age. He had a neighborhood best friend, Doug, who would accompany him everywhere. Scott liked to speed on his Yamaha motorcycle on dirt paths with Doug holding on for his life. We all listened to rock music in the early 1980s, and Scott idolized Jim Morrison of the Doors. It was around this time that I started to notice a big change in my brother. Normally our school made an effort to separate twins into different sections, and trigonometry was the first class that Scott and I had together. I remember glancing over at Scott and instead of seeing him concentrating on the lecture and taking notes, I noticed that his eyes were glazed over and he was often staring out the window. I thought to myself, "What is he doing?" He clearly was not paying attention to the teacher during class; instead he seemed to have been starting to withdraw and descend into a scary and strange new world.

I also began to realize something was wrong with Scott after waking up one night and hearing him crying to my mother about how he felt bullied in school and that he had no friends. I could certainly relate to his feelings since I also found high school to be a difficult time. My mom thought a change of scene would solve our problems, so Scott, my mom, and I all moved to a new town. I started a new high school, and my brother took his high school courses at a community college. My mom helped Scott buy his first car so he could drive to college. Mom also helped Scott obtain a summer job with the engineering department at Mobil Chemical where she worked, while I worked at McDonald's serving up Big Macs and fries with a friendly smile. My brother was so excited and at first loved the change; he excelled in the company of scientists and was considered a "boy-genius," writing computer programs that helped regulate shipments out of the plant. Scott felt like he had found his ideal job working with the engineering department since he loved math and science, and he imagined himself as an engineer some day working in a laboratory.

All of my brother's dreams came to a screeching halt, however, when he lost control of his thoughts and feelings. I remember one day hearing the familiar Doors music coming from his bedroom so I thought I would go in to listen and spend some time with him. I knocked and received no response. I opened the door only to find all kinds of hand-colored paper pyramids and triangles strategically positioned around the room, some on top of his record turnstile, and clothing hangers that were bent into antenna shapes. I remember thinking, "Wow, this is all very strange." But, it was not strange to Scott. To him there was a perfectly reasonable explanation for it all; this arrangement was designed by Scott to enable him to receive special messages through the air that were meant only for him. Of course, this made the whole situation appear even weirder to me.

I also remember sharing our birthday cake when we turned 17 years old. I thought everything was okay until Scott announced to our mom and grandparents that I was the daughter of the devil. We all thought that surely Scott was not serious and that he was saying things to get a reaction from us, but he continued to insist, and he explained that he knew of the very dark and evil things that were occurring in the world, his sentences losing meaning as he fused one paranoid and bizarre thought into another. As Scott's 17-year-old twin, his behavior frightened me. I did not understand it and I found myself not wanting to stay at home; I found every excuse to go out in the evening. This left my mom at home to try to help Scott think clearly and to see reality. Unfortunately, this approach did not work, and my brother turned on my mom one night, hurting her physically by knocking her against a wall and threatening to harm her. I was at home that night when my mom screamed for me to help and call the police. It was horrific to see the police take my twin brother away from home, but it was the only thing my mom and I could do. My mom went to the police station, and my brother was so psychotic that he claimed our mom was not his mother; in his "reality," Yoko Ono was his mother. He said many other things that did not make sense, and the police recognized that my brother seriously needed psychiatric evaluation.

At that time, during the early 1980s, my brother was placed in a large state psychiatric hospital. He looked much like a young scared boy among a ward full of older people, some of whom were pacing, drooling, or rocking back and forth and appearing only half human. It was a terrible shock to see him in a stark white room and even worse to see him struggle with medication. He was placed on a high dose of first-generation antipsychotic medication that made him feel very uncomfortable. My mom and I later discovered that his experience with antipsychotic medicine was the most horrible experience of his life, and Scott explained that he would rather die than have to go through his experience at the psychiatric ward again. When he returned home to live with my grandparents, I remember that he would pace the floor, and eventually he developed what we were told was tardive dyskinesia, uncontrollable movements of his mouth and tongue. Seeing my twin brother suffer with his illness and the horrible side effects of his inadequate treatment motivated me to dedicate my life to research the underlying cause of this devastating disorder, ultimately to develop better and more rational treatments. I knew that I wanted to try to understand the brain on the cellular and molecular level, but I did not even know the field of neuroscience existed when I made this commitment after high school. So, I studied both biology and psychology in college, went on to graduate school, and then later postdoctoral training, eventually establishing my own research laboratory.

In the late 1980s, the most prominent theory of schizophrenia centered on the dopamine system, but I had always viewed schizophrenia as a developmental disorder since I had grown up with a "normal" twin brother who eventually changed into someone I could not recognize during our adolescent years. I experienced similar biologic changes and social challenges as a teenager as Scott did, but Scott's life took a dramatically different course. I wanted to understand if the typical changes that occur during brain maturation did not occur properly in the brains of people who suffered from schizophrenia, particularly as I began to realize that my brother's story was common. Many men who develop schizophrenia first experience their symptoms during late adolescence or early adulthood after a relatively normal childhood.

So, my quest to understand schizophrenia and develop better treatments was born in the living room of my childhood home in the early 1980s. By the time I had my own research program on schizophrenia, my brother was receiving the newer second-generation antipsychotic medication. Scott finally appeared to improve, and he began feeling much better. However, he still spent the majority of his time in his bedroom, studying math and science books or reading novels. He did manage to get out of our childhood home and helped elderly neighbors by bringing them to their doctor appointments, shoveling snow from their sidewalks, and delivering "meals on wheels" to shut-ins. He even traveled to England with me and my husband. Scott was able to tour a country he had only dreamed of visiting. He also attended photography classes at the community college and chemistry classes taught by some of my former teachers at Keuka College with the hope of assisting me in my research laboratory some day. Although he felt the social stress of the classroom interfered with his learning and test taking, he was able to complete three semesters. I bought a house where Scott intended to come to live with me some day. Although Scott was improved psychologically from the newer medication, he had excessive weight gain and suffered from diabetes, which can be common side effects of antipsychotic medication.

I was attracted to lead a schizophrenia research program in Sydney, Australia, and although it was far away from my brother, I had an opportunity to double my research team, develop a department, and lead a team of researchers focused on the developmental neurobiology of schizophrenia. We hope to make progress toward developing new medications that will further improve the lives of people with schizophrenia. Although this time is professionally exciting for me, I am personally very saddened because my twin brother has recently passed away and I miss him dearly. I loved Scott so much, and I wish I could have done more to improve his life. I hope you find this book helpful in better understanding schizophrenia. One day I hope we will have answers to prevent and cure this terrible disease.

A diagnosis of a disease such as schizophrenia, often thought to be "all in your mind," leaves patients and their loved ones filled with questions and fears. This makes a book such as the second edition of *100 Questions & Answers About Schizophrenia* very important. Dr. DeLisi's book fills the need for comprehending a misunderstood illness such as schizophrenia. Using this book as a resource will provide the knowledge that is necessary to cope with the diagnosis of mental illness. Sadly, my brother lost his battle with this disease, but others may not. The psychic pain of mental illness is often as hard to bear as the physical pain of a cancer. However, there is hope for a positive outcome in the future made possible by continuing research such as that done by Dr. DeLisi, myself, and our colleagues.

Cyndi Shannon-Weickert, PhD
Sydney, Australia

A Nurse's Perspective

I turned my head away, embarrassed for the stranger I did not even know. I started to talk to my husband because I did not want him to see the person walking on the sidewalk. The man had many layers of clothing on and was filthy. He appeared to be having a whole conversation with himself. As a young child, my mother had told me to stay away from "those people" because they were "crazy" and may hurt me.

One night, after turning my head away from "those crazy people" for several years, my whole life and understanding of them changed. I started a job working the night shift on a 28-bed admitting psychiatric unit, and it was time to face my fears. As I locked the door behind me, I wondered if this was something I was capable of doing, if I would ever stop being afraid. Twenty years later I am still caring for this population as a registered nurse, and I can't imagine doing anything else. I am no longer afraid and now can see that I was afraid because I did not understand mental illness.

Providing care for a patient with schizophrenia can be very challenging. By the time people are admitted to a psychiatric ward in a hospital facility, they are usually extremely decompensated. They may be psychotic, paranoid, delusional, and experiencing auditory or visual hallucinations. All of these symptoms have an impact on how the nurse will care for the patient and his or her family.

For the past 20 years, I have cared for not only the mentally ill patient but also for those who are part of another special population, the United States veterans. I have worked in inpatient as well as outpatient settings with veterans. It is one of the most rewarding opportunities I have ever had, as well as one of the most challenging.

Caring for the mentally ill veteran population brings many challenges. Veterans are different because of the training they received while in the service. They are trained to kill and have an in-depth understanding of self-defense techniques that the general population does not possess. This does not mean that the veteran population is more violent than the general population. It just means that there is a special caution you use when approaching or being approached by a psychotic veteran. Not all mentally ill people are violent, and not all violent people are mentally ill. Most of the veterans I have worked with are kind and compassionate people who would never harm anyone, so they struggle with the voices that are telling them to harm themselves or others. Many choose to harm themselves rather than others and it is well documented that the veteran population has a significantly higher suicide rate than the general public. The environment in the VA system is in constant flux in an attempt to provide a safe environment for the suicidal patient. Many patients with schizophrenia who harm themselves do so as a result of the voices that are telling them to or as an attempt to escape the voices and the mental anguish. As a nurse, I ask patients on a daily basis if they are having pain, and there is nothing more heartbreaking than when they say, "Yes, in my head." Many times I have felt helpless as a nurse to alleviate their pain. Many attempt suicide to escape this pain.

Frequently the patients I treat are paranoid. A lot of the paranoia in the veteran population centers on the government and its agencies, such as the FBI or CIA. They express thoughts that the government is trying to kill them because of information they have obtained while in the service and believe the FBI or CIA are looking for them. Many believe "chips" have been placed in their body by the government so that they can be monitored and their activities followed. I have seen a patient pull out his own teeth because his delusion is so strong that there is a device in his teeth to track him.

One of the things I find the most frustrating about caring for a schizophrenic person is dealing with the paranoid belief that medications and food are being poisoned. As a nurse, you know that patients must take in nourishment, yet they refuse all you offer. The problem is how do you get them to take the medications and food when they are so paranoid? Without the medications, they will not improve, and without fluids, they may become dehydrated. I find that it becomes a situation of negotiations. Most of the patients want something, whether it is a cigarette or to go off the hospital ward with staff; at times, this is what the staff uses to bargain with. Many patients will bargain with the staff that they will take their medications if they are allowed to smoke. Staff is aware that sometimes the only way to get patients to take nourishment is to lessen the paranoia by use of medications. What is the best ethical decision? Do you leave the patients alone with their paranoia, which ultimately results in forcing medication upon them, or do you negotiate, which is the less intrusive method?

While there are many frustrating moments when caring for the patient with schizoprhenia, there are so many pleasures and rewarding times. One of my responsibilities in outpatient care was providing case management for the severely mentally ill. It was my job to assist veterans in staying in the community and decreasing the number of hospitalizations. I would teach them to grocery shop, help them maintain a bank account and pay their bills, make sure they went to their doctor's appointments, and ensure that they took their medications as prescribed. It was a very rewarding and fulfilling job to see the patients in the community functioning at their maximum ability.

With this position also came the opportunity for me to witness the stigma that comes with a mental health diagnosis. I have seen how the mentally ill are treated in society, how people laugh behind their back and even sometimes to their face, how people look the other way, like I used to, out of fear and misunderstanding. I have seen people treat them like they are second-class citizens who do not belong in society. I was once with a patient in a facility for a medical appointment, and when the elevator stopped and we got on, all the people looked at each other and walked off like they might catch something from the patient.

Every day I go to work not only thankful that I have a job but also feeling blessed that I am privileged to work with the mentally ill population.

Catherine Giasson, BSN, RN
Nurse Manager at the Veterans Administration, Boston Health Care System in Chronic and Acute Psychiatry*

---

*Disclaimer: The views expressed in this foreword are those of the author and do not reflect the official policy of the Department of the Army, Department of Defense, VA, or U.S. Government.

Note from the Author

The inspiring story of Scott as written by his twin sister, Cyndi, one of my colleagues, exemplifies how typical a life someone with schizophrenia begins with. Until early adulthood, they have the interests, hopes, and aspirations of so many youth of their generation. Although Scott had many advantages when he first became ill, too often other patients are lost to treatment in the current U.S. mental healthcare system that is governed by insurance policies and overworked caregivers. Adequate intensive follow-up care is sometimes not given to those who clearly need it, particularly early in the illness course after first being diagnosed, partly because they do not recognize their need for it. Thus, patients can slip by with warning signs unnoticed. It is often left to families to take on this responsibility of knowing early enough when their relative is slipping into another episode of illness. Unfortunately, some patients are not lucky enough to have family members who stay supportive during the periods of evolving "strange" behavior such as that described by Dr. Shannon-Weickert.*

The perspective here of one nurse, Catherine, who has dedicated her life to helping people with mental illness, states clearly both the frustrations and rewards that come with her work, a service that is too often unnoticed by the public in general, families of patients, and the community of professionals. Many of the patients she sees are at the other end of the spectrum, those patients who are already chronic and have gone through multiple hospitalizations and treatment regimes and are often abandoned by their families and other support networks. They are considered "end stage" by too many mental care workers who by this time have given up hope for rehabilitating them. I call these patients "the forgotten" because too often the focus is on the beginning stages of illness, i.e., early detection and treatment both in the research and clinical worlds. However, the quality of life of those who have had persistent illness for many years should not be ignored. This is an illness

*All too often, even when they have this support, they are lost to suicide, as happened with Scott.

that is not likely to be irradicated for years to come. Thus, we all continue to work toward achieving public recognition that schizophrenia is a medical disease and not some scary unknown behavior to stigmatize, and that parity for mental illness in the healthcare system is necessary for improving the quality of care for these patients so that no one patient or family of a patient needlessly suffers. In addition, we continue to focus on developing new and better treatments, so that ultimately the "end stage" described in these "forgotten" ones that exists today on the chronic hospital psychiatric wards worldwide will be preventable.

Lynn E. DeLisi, MD
Brockton, Massachusetts

Introduction

I knew that I would somehow do something to inform the public of what I consider to be the facts about schizophrenia when my daughter came home from high school in the 1980s saying that her health class teacher described schizophrenia as a "split personality." At the time, I had already been treating patients with schizophrenia and performing research about this disorder for several years. I knew this statement could not be further from the truth. Schizophrenia has long been known not to be a Jekyll and Hyde type of condition, yet what we long knew as psychiatrists was somehow not being communicated to the public. When Bleuler coined the term "schizophrenia" in 1911, he erroneously used the Latin for "split mind." What he meant was that there was a "split"—or inconsistency—between the affect and emotions, thought and speech, and perhaps perception and reality. Unfortunately what we name a condition can have repercussions for many years into the future. The Japanese may now take the lead in changing the name of this illness to something more reflective of its biology, as they accumulate supportive data to suggest that a name alone can induce the stigma that accompanies a disorder such as schizophrenia.

This term has continued over the years to describe a psychiatric disorder that is very heterogeneous in its expression, clinical course, and biology. Schizophrenia has had an unusual course in history. At the turn of the twentieth century, patients with these symptoms were shunned by society and isolated in large, gated multi-building complexes called psychiatric hospitals or institutions, often being committed there by relatives and staying for years or for life. At World War II, the Nazi extermination policy began with a focus on patients in psychiatric hospitals, as they were deemed unfit to live and use a share of limited national resources. Many psychiatrists even played terrible roles in facilitating these policies because of their lack of understanding of the biology and inheritance of this disorder.

It was only in the late 1960s, when neuroleptic medications were accepted as the treatment of choice and marked improvement in behavior could be seen, that patients were rehabilitated back into the community. Slowly the public institutions were emptied, and residences sprang up within towns for patients who were stabilized and were treatable on an outpatient basis in the community. Periodically, questions about the nature of this illness resurface when someone with schizophrenia is in the news for having performed a violent act toward an innocent person; then the prudence of releasing some patients prematurely from long-term hospital commitment is questioned.

One such famous case was John Hinckley, Jr., the young man who shot former President Reagan and one of his cabinet members (James Brady, who was permanently disabled subsequent to this attack). Of course, many more people who do not have a diagnosis of schizophrenia commit violent acts than those with the diagnosis, but nevertheless, unpredictable behavior is a frightening hallmark of unstabilized or undertreated symptoms of schizophrenia, particularly of the paranoid type. These types of behaviors, plus the bizarreness and inappropriateness of some of the symptoms, lead to a dire social consequence that has implications for not only whether someone seeks appropriate treatment but also for how someone with this diagnosis is viewed by people with whom he or she interacts socially, professionally, and legally. These characteristics lead to the stigma that has been formed about schizophrenia over the years.

Unfortunately, physicians, because of the stigma attached to the disorder, will often delay making a schizophrenia diagnosis and will then likely cause more damage by initially assuring parents that their son or daughter will "grow out of it." They will instead label the emotional difficulties as an "adjustment reaction," which requires no medication but simply observation and psychotherapy over time. The harm is that we now know it is likely that early pharmacologic treatment may prevent the severe, chronic, debilitating form of this illness.

The stigmatization associated with this illness extends into further aspects of life. Insurance companies do not treat schizophrenia as a medical illness that needs treatment in the same way as pneumonia, for instance, or other ailments that originate below the head. Employers would likely eliminate anyone who wrote on a job application that he or she was in the past or is currently diagnosed with schizophrenia. Families keep secret that one of their relatives is afflicted because the stigma may contribute to a potential mate's reluctance to marry into such a family. As with a history of depression, having had schizophrenia in one's past is used against those rare individuals who recover, so that they are unlikely to ever hold a government office or to succeed in ways that they could have were it not for their diagnosis.

Nevertheless, many famous and creative figures have been said to have schizophrenia or at least a psychotic illness that at times was certainly indistinguishable from schizophrenia. Among them are musicians (such as Brian Wilson from the Beach Boys), artists (Van Gogh), Nobel Prize winners (John Nash), kings (Christian VII of Denmark in the late 1700s), and historical figures such as Joan of Arc. They contrast at an extreme with other individuals diagnosed with this disorder, such as the Unabomber or the Yorkshire Ripper. Famous movies have depicted people with schizophrenia for decades, from the early horrors in *The Snake Pit*, to *One Flew Over the Cuckoo's Nest*, to *I Never Promised You a Rose Garden*, and most recently, *A Beautiful Mind* and *Changeling*. The latter film was particularly damaging. In it, Angelina Jolie plays a single mother whose child disappears. The police are less than sympathetic toward her and ultimately put her away in a mental institution, where she is treated for speaking out as if she had symptoms of schizophrenia and is met with a lack of compassion and nastiness from the nurses, orderlies, and doctors. Any potential psychiatric patient who sees this 2008 movie will likely not seek help for fear of being mistreated.

Although some people aid in quelling the stigma surrounding this illness, others point fingers at people with schizophrenia, considering them peculiar and using the words *cuckoo*, *nuts*, or *loco* to describe their thoughts and behavior. Most people who stigmatize people with schizophrenia know little about the scientific basis for this illness and whether their prejudices make practical sense. This book is designed to refute the basis for the stigma surrounding schizophrenia and to provide the public with a glimpse of what it is like to have this disorder, what causes it, how it can be treated, and how to live a productive life when you or a family member has schizophrenia.

Lynn E. DeLisi, MD

PART ONE

The Illness and Its Characteristics

What is schizophrenia?

How is schizophrenia different from bipolar disease (or manic depression)?

What is meant by "positive" and "negative" symptoms?

More . . .

Schizophrenia

Characterized by social withdrawal, disorganized patterns of thinking and speaking, multiple delusions, and hallucinations, accompanied in varying degrees by other emotional, behavioral, or intellectual disturbances.

DSM-IV

Diagnostic and Statistical Manual of Mental Disorders IV, developed by leading clinical psychiatrists in the United States for systematically evaluating psychiatric patients and assigning diagnoses to groups of symptoms.

Delusion

A false belief based on faulty judgment about one's environment.

Hallucination

The experience of something from any of the five senses that is not occurring in reality.

Prodrome

An early or premonitory symptom of a disease.

Residual

Having some nonspecific symptoms (usually negative symptoms) but no longer active psychotic ones.

"By New Year's Day . . . Nash's behavior had become more and more peculiar. He was irritable and hypersensitive one minute, eerily withdrawn the next. He complained that he knew that something was going on and that he was being bugged. Also, he was staying up nights writing strange letters to the United Nations. One night he had painted black spots all over our [sic] *bedroom wall."*

As told to Sylvia Nasar in an interview with the wife of John Nash, Nobel Laureate, (1994), 1998

1. What is schizophrenia?

The American Psychiatric Association defines **schizophrenia** in its ***Diagnostic and Statistical Manual of Mental Disorders IV* (*DSM-IV*)** as a disorder with active symptoms for at least 1 month, consisting of **delusions**, **hallucinations**, disorganized speech, grossly disorganized/bizarre behavior, and/or a lack of organized speech, activity, or emotions. Usually at least two of these sets of symptoms are present. The illness, with a **prodromal** stage prior to diagnosis and a **residual** stage after treatment (both having some often nonspecific behavioral symptoms), lasts at least 6 months with continuous signs of some disturbance. During this period, an individual with schizophrenia is clearly considered impaired in his or her ability to perform at work, attend school, or participate in social activities in a productive way.

The hallucinations of schizophrenia are most often auditory, although visual, olfactory, and tactile hallucinations have been described as well. The latter, however, are more often due to substance abuse (alcohol or street drugs) than schizophrenia when they predominate.

The auditory hallucinations that distinguish schizophrenia are not just sounds. They are words spoken aloud as if someone else is actually speaking them, although no one is there. The words can derive from one person who is or is not recognized by the individual and who is commenting in some way on the hearer's behavior. They also can be perceived as multiple voices talking about the hearer, usually in a frightening or derogatory manner. Sometimes the hallucinations have been occurring for years before any other symptoms and go unrecognized by the individual as anything that is abnormal or not happening to everyone. Many times, when severe, they intrude into the person's life and daily activities. The patient can be found actually responding to the voices as if in conversation. Without experience, any examiner might have difficulty imagining what hallucinations are like.

The word *delusion* is certainly common, but the delusions of schizophrenia can sometimes be characteristic. Many are bizarre to the normal person. For example, patients frequently mention feeling that some unknown force is controlling their actions or emotions or that they can see objects in the environment with new meaning. Similarly, they may be watching television or a movie and feel that the people on the screen are giving them special messages. Common environmental situations, such as water dripping from a faucet, take on a new, magical meaning. Patients may describe feeling that parts of their body are not their own, as well as feeling like they are actors on the "stage of life" and not "real" people. Other common symptoms are the perceived ability to mind read or the feeling that other people know their thoughts, as if they are spoken on a loudspeaker. Patients with schizophrenia are suspicious that people are harming them (e.g., by food poisoning) or that a complicated plot by the government against them is occurring.

Paranoia

Suspicions that other people are doing harmful things to oneself such as watching or observing oneself unnecessarily. This is a general mistrust of other people that can develop into extreme delusions.

These latter **paranoid** delusions may be accompanied by delusions of grandeur (thinking that one has extraordinary powers or abilities that are in reality not possessed) and hyperreligiosity that becomes delusional ("knowing" that God has singled one out for a special mission or simply controls and dictates all of one's actions). I once had a patient who knew he would "be president of the United States" because "God had told him." This was, however, someone who had been barely an average student throughout school and thought that London, England, was in the midwestern United States! I have had another patient who consistently confers with God for every daily decision he must make and when asked a question by a nurse, will hold up his hand, say "just a minute" and walk off into a corner to confer with God first before answering.

Most psychiatrists today would agree that schizophrenia is defined by at least three separate sets of symptoms:

1. Positive symptoms, which include hallucinations and delusions.
2. Negative symptoms, which include a general appearance of being flat (without much emotion), called "flat affect"; withdrawal; a lack of much speech, at least speech that says anything; and slow movements and the appearance of slow thought.
3. A set of symptoms related to general disorganization (i.e., speech that is mixed or not getting to the point and behavioral disorganization). These symptoms are now considered a separate cluster, defined as **disorganization syndrome**.

Disorganization syndrome

A set of symptoms related to general disorganization (i.e., speech that is mixed or not getting to the point and behavioral disorganization). These symptoms are now considered a separate cluster.

Subtypes of schizophrenia and different types of related diagnoses exist as well. The paranoid subtype involves delusions and hallucinations more heavily, rather than any disorganization, and the symptoms are often, but not always, paranoid in nature. The disorganized subtype has most prominently the disorganization symptoms already mentioned. The catatonic subtype focuses predominantly on motor and speech changes that are either excessive or deficient. The undifferentiated subtype is generally a mixture of the others, with one type not being most prominent. Finally, the residual subtype is one in which the patient has become stabilized and no longer has the delusions and hallucinations but still does not seem normal and has many so-called negative symptoms (appearing withdrawn, speaking minimally, lacking initiative, etc.) that have not resolved.

2. Is schizophrenia a split personality?

The word *schizophrenia* is clearly a misnomer. Eugene Bleuler, who coined this term back in the early part of the twentieth century, did so because he saw an abnormal "split" between the outward affect of the patient and his or her emotions and a split between thought, speech, and affect. The split is actually due to an underlying misconnection of brain functional activity.

A split personality is quite a rare syndrome whereby a person assumes different identities; an environmental trigger initiates this switch. Usually these identities have been manifest because of traumatic events, such as sexual abuse, that took place in the individual's childhood and that have been extremely stressful to acknowledge. These individuals may benefit from intense psychotherapy over the years but are in no way similar clinically or biologically to people with schizophrenia.

Not only is the term *schizophrenia* misleading, but it leads to stigmatization of people; many well-meaning people use the abbreviated "schizo" to describe anyone who behaves in a strange way or seems to be inconsistent or "split." Some people are starting movements in different parts of the world to change the name of this disorder to something with a more meaningful connotation. This change remains in the future.

3. What are the first signs of this illness? How do I know whether I (or my relative) have schizophrenia?

The following case illustrates the essence of this question:

Maryanne was a first-year medical student who received an educational loan that covered only the subsidized housing development in which she was forced to live. She took a job as a waitress in a nearby bar on hours when she was not on student patient call in the evening. She gained support from a group of same-sex classmates and would often study with them in afternoons after class or during lunch breaks. Tension was high during exams, and classmate support was often emotionally helpful. Occasionally marijuana was passed from student to student during mass cramming sessions and occasionally, after smoking heavily, Maryanne would complain about other people and become anxious about some private things she refused to discuss. Laurie, a fellow classmate, noticed at some point that Maryanne was missing classes, occasionally at first and then more frequently. Finally, she and three other friends made the trip across town to Maryanne's apartment. The lights were dim, and at first their knocks went unheard. Chanting was overheard by the girls, however, and thus they persisted. Eventually, Maryanne came to the door inappropriately dressed in Muslim robes. Candles glowed in a circle surrounding her living room, and food and other items were scattered across the floor. Maryanne explained that she had taken up meditating and had converted to a Muslim sect, reciting some verses from the Koran. She assured her friends that she was fine but preferred to stay home that day. Eventually, when school administrators noticed her absence, she was called in and required to attend psychotherapy in order to return to school. Instead, she dropped out of school and disappeared.

Eventually, she was unemployed and lost her apartment. She became homeless for a time and received a small note in the local paper when she finally committed suicide by attempting a bizarre baptism in the ocean.

Stories such as Maryanne's are too common. Although they luckily do not all lead to suicide, many do lead to a cessation of normal life and, for young adults, a loss of the potential that the future held. Often relatives and close friends are unaware of why the individual is wary of confiding in anyone and remains reclusive or hard to find. The person who is developing schizophrenia rarely has any insight that he or she is ill and thus does not admit to anyone the stressful thoughts and perceptions occurring, despite their disturbing nature, and does not seek help. Those who are close—friends and relatives—may notice a change in behavior and emotional responses; however, they do not know that the affected person is having hallucinations and delusionary thoughts unless the person says things that sound bizarre or that clearly cannot be true. Often, particularly when of a paranoid nature, these things are kept to oneself. Families, if intact, after recognizing problems will rally to the support of the ill individual but often do not think the person needs professional help unless the behavior becomes extreme. Once they do obtain help for their sick relative, as time goes by they are eventually depleted of funds and frustrated by the lack of community and legal support to aid their relative. Parents eventually become resigned to care for these children permanently, but as they age, they worry about who will care for their child after they are gone.

Psychiatric researchers continuously debate how best to predict whether a schizophrenic-like illness is likely to occur. It would be useful to find clear predictors that can distinguish the symptoms of illness from the variation in functioning and the "ups and downs" of stages of life experiences, particularly in adolescence. No such predictors, however, have clearly been found. The key probably has to do with change from one's usual functioning (i.e., withdrawal from friendships, peculiar statements that are not true, and a change in organization of behavior and speech). Work and school activities change for the worse and an overall troubled withdrawal of the individual becomes apparent to those with whom he or she interacts. This individual may be heard talking to himself or herself or making untrue or bizarre statements about other people or events. These symptoms often accelerate to the point that the individual can behave in an inappropriate or harmful manner (such as undressing in public or walking down the middle of a highway). In other instances, the individual will perform impulsive and aggressive acts without understanding the consequence of such actions. At this point, the police are called, and the individual is brought to either jail or a psychiatric emergency room. Obviously, it is beneficial if early signs can be recognized and treated before they accelerate to a dangerous situation.

In general, schizophrenia develops gradually, on average over about a 2-year period in an adolescent or young adult. Behavioral changes—such as withdrawing socially, a noticeable decline in academic performance, irritability, or what appears as **depression**—are first noticed by close friends or family. The individuals may also be found sleeping either too much or too little and are periodically agitated. These things might eventually lead parents to consult a family physician about their child. Parents might be told that adolescent turmoil or adjustment problems are the cause. Most physicians delay making a diagnosis of schizophrenia, particularly if the patient does not admit to clear auditory hallucinations and bizarre delusions. The stigma of having this disorder is great and the notion that it is like a "cancer of the mind" that lasts a lifetime is a "death sentence" that no physician wants to give unless he or she can no longer avoid it. The message to a parent may simply be that "he or she will grow out of it." Frequent follow-up, however, should be instituted in these cases.

Depression

Profound sadness lasting day and night, accompanied by physical symptoms, such as loss of appetite, loss of sleep, and slowness in movements and speech. If the condition continues as long as 2 weeks without relief and interferes with a person's ability to function, it is then called major depression.

The stigma of having this disorder is great and the notion that it is like a "cancer of the mind" that lasts a lifetime is a "death sentence" that no physician wants to give unless he or she can no longer avoid it.

The patient may eventually admit to clear symptoms, which gives the opportunity for early treatment and possible prevention of the severe chronic form of the illness. The typical case, however, is a young person who has done something that is clearly bizarre and so harmful, either to himself or herself or to others, that the police or a psychiatric crisis unit is called for help. In at least half of the cases in several countries, some kind of street drug use may be acutely responsible or may at least contribute to the bizarre and harmful behavior when it becomes a crisis.

Many first-episode patients, after being treated and having the symptoms resolve, conclude that drug use was the cause and that they will be okay as long as they abstain from drugs (see Part 6 for a more detailed discussion of drug abuse). This assumption, however, is in many cases false. The drugs may have initiated the disease that might have eventually occurred regardless at a later time under some other stress. The danger is that the patient will assume that he or she does not need the **neuroleptic** medication prescribed as long as street drugs are not taken again. The medications and treatment given during the acute episode are terminated, and the patient eventually comes back to the hospital in a more serious relapse of symptoms that are generally more difficult to suppress with medication. The patient who terminates his or her first treatment without being integrated into the chronic care system is most likely to commit suicide.

Neuroleptic

Any medication that will cause catalepsy when given to animals. This name is used to label all drugs that have an effect on reducing the symptoms of schizophrenia. They are sometimes known as the "major tranquilizers."

As can be seen, stigma both by the general public and by physicians who diagnose and treat is a serious problem that will need to be conquered if this disorder is to be identified early and treated aggressively before chronic deterioration sets in.

4. Is being "schizophreniform" the same as having schizophrenia?

In **schizophreniform** disorder, a patient has all the symptoms of schizophrenia, but the symptoms resolve in less than 6 months without residual symptoms. Generally, this person was functioning very well and acutely developed symptoms that resolved relatively quickly with or without medication. However, someone may initially be diagnosed as schizophreniform, and after 6 months the illness evolves into a clear diagnosis of schizophrenia—that is, some symptoms remain, even if medications are effective in suppressing most symptoms, and the doctor feels it is in the best interest of the patient to continue on medication. The majority of

Schizophreniform

Having the symptoms of schizophrenia, but too early in the course of illness to tell whether the symptoms are of a schizophrenia illness.

people who have a diagnosis of schizophreniform disorder eventually are diagnosed with schizophrenia.

5. What does it mean to have a "schizotypal personality"?

There are mild forms of schizophrenia that sometimes are present in family members of people who have schizophrenia. Sometimes they are just referred to as the spectrum disorders and other times as schizotypal. This term refers to specific traits that make one stand out and are often thought of as peculiar. Such traits may include:

- Speech that is too formal for the specific conversation (stilted)
- Speech that is unfocused and rambling
- Belief in ESP, horoscopes, or strange superstitions
- Strange feelings and perceptions from time to time
- Feelings of paranoia and suspicions of others beyond reason
- Indifference to having friends and socializing

These traits may be stable over time and characteristic of the person and may perhaps interfere with leading a "normal" life or result in the individual living alone in peculiar or bizarre circumstances. For example, everyone has at one time or another noticed an acquaintance or someone in the neighborhood who appears peculiar, who hoards stacks of newspapers piled high in his or her house, as well as collections of other objects; or one might see or hear about another neighbor with nine cats who is known to live in the dark with curtains drawn during the day.

Many of the traits of schizotypal personality can also be interchanged with paranoid and schizoid personality disorders, the former mainly a disorder of unreasonable or distorted suspicion about others and the latter a disorder of social withdrawal and a preference to be by oneself. Each disorder emphasizes different types of traits, but these traits are frequently related and all present in the same individual.

6. What is schizoaffective disorder?

Schizoaffective disorder is a related diagnosis to both schizophrenia and bipolar disorder and may be the same as either of these illnesses in its biologic origins. A patient with this disorder has all the symptoms of schizophrenia but also has significantly overlapping symptoms of depression, **manic behavior**, or both. Depression is generally defined as feeling very sad emotionally, perhaps to the point of having suicidal ideas or actions, with loss of weight and sleep often as a result. Manic behavior, on the other hand, is defined by feeling excessively elated and cheery with very fast speech and thoughts; individuals in a manic state may perform bizarre and risky acts and may behave in an agitated manner. Grandiose delusions are also part of this syndrome.

Schizoaffective

Having prominent symptoms both of schizophrenia and of depression and/or mania.

Manic behavior

Characterized by a rapid pace in both speech and movements, euphoria or irritability, needing little sleep, impulsive and reckless behavior, sometimes accompanied by grandiose delusions of having special abilities and powers, and auditory hallucinations.

Interestingly, psychiatrists generally differ in whether they would diagnose someone with schizophrenia or schizoaffective disorder, as well as any of the subtypes of schizophrenia, and over the course of illness, these diagnoses in one individual seem to change. Similarly, they disagree whether someone with schizoaffective disorder should at some times be diagnosed with **bipolar affective disorder** (also called manic depression). Thus, patients who are sometimes diagnosed with schizoaffective disorder may be seen by some psychiatrists as having only schizophrenia but may be seen by others as having bipolar disorder too.

Bipolar affective disorder

A psychiatric condition characterized by mood swings that occur episodically. Sometimes, particularly when very "high" (manic), people with bipolar disorder can have many of the characteristic positive symptoms of schizophrenia.

One view is that a biologic continuum likely exists between all these diagnoses. The extremes and classical cases of each are more consistently diagnosable among psychiatrists, but the vast majority fall somewhere in the middle, schizoaffective category being the middle. They can either be called schizophrenia-spectrum disorder or they can be classified and treated by the symptoms that occur, rather than the category of diagnosis. It may be that the underlying biology of what appear to be different illnesses is the same. However, the clinical manifestations may vary in different individuals, from a very disorganized schizophrenia-like degenerative illness to a cyclic episode of **psychotic** symptoms with normality in between—the so-called "unitary psychosis" (Crow, 1990). Alternatively, there may be several biologic causes, but their clinical manifestations may cross over the traditional diagnostic boundaries that psychiatry has established. When we have definitely determined the related biologic underpinnings (such as genes or their expression) for aspects of schizophrenia, it is anticipated that entirely different diagnostic categories may be developed that will then reflect the illness biology more directly.

Psychotic

A condition defined by losing touch with reality or having delusions (i.e., false beliefs) and hallucinations. Psychotic individuals often exhibit bizarre and risky behavior and do not seem to be aware that they are doing anything unusual.

7. How is schizophrenia different from bipolar disease (or manic depression)?

Although, as mentioned in the previous question, some research psychiatrists believe that a biologic continuum exists between the extremes of these two disorders, there are differences. Many people with bipolar disorder can lead a normal, productive, and very creative life after their mood is stabilized. In fact, before the full-blown illness, these individuals may be high achievers and model citizens in their community; thus, once the symptoms develop into a crisis, those around them are surprised and bewildered that they somehow missed that something was wrong.

Take, for example, the Boston "Craigslist Killer," recently notorious in the U.S. national news. This individual was a medical student, a star by all criteria, who was socially very well liked and academically performing very well. The only indication of anything wrong was that one person described him as "having mood swings." However, given the normal stresses in this young man's life, mood changes would not be unusual. What was unusual was his sudden bizarre and risky behavior, meeting massage therapists in hotels, hoarding their underwear, and finally shooting one with a gun that he had kept in a hollowed-out *Gray's Anatomy* text. One could speculate from reading descriptions in the news that this man was not a usual criminal, but rather someone who clearly developed the onset of a psychotic disorder, likely a bipolar disorder, that unfortunately was not checked before his behavior became harmful to others.

This story, although an extreme that made news headlines, is all too frequent. Nevertheless, after stabilization on medication and after such a manic episode, providing that medication is continued, individuals with this condition appear not to lose their original potential for functioning. Cognitive abilities are not impaired, as they are in schizophrenia, and individuals with bipolar disorder may be able to go back to their normal lives if they have not committed a crime during the acute stage of illness such as the medical student mentioned here. There are also, however, more severe cases of bipolar disorder with several frequent hospitalizations that eventually are indistinguishable from schizophrenia.

Premorbid

The time period before any symptoms of a disorder, including subtle signs, have developed.

Thus, both the **premorbid** state and the outcome constitute the difference between schizophrenia and bipolar disorder, although some of the symptoms and the biology may be similar. Schizophrenia is more often thought of as a **neurodevelopmental** disorder with a poor premorbid adjustment socially and academically in childhood (although not always). Prebipolar individuals are indistinguishable from others in those earlier years.

Neurodevelopment

Happening during the growth and formation of different structures of the brain. This may be prenatally, during childhood, or even through adolescence and early adulthood.

Much biologic research comparing the biology of these two disorders needs to be performed. Although many of the brain structural changes present in schizophrenia have been found in bipolar disorder, severe bipolar disorder with psychotic features (such as hallucinations and delusions) appears to show these changes. Some of these differences and similarities are detailed in a book published by Maneros and Angst in 2000 (*Bipolar Disorders: 100 Years After Manic Depressive Insanity*), two researchers who have focused over the years on these issues.

8. Is it possible to hear voices that are not there and not be ill?

Recently, reports of surveys of the general non-treatment-seeking population conclude that auditory hallucinations and various forms of delusions are common. In fact, the investigators of these studies report that psychotic experiences are present in anywhere from 5%–20% of the general population. This statement needs to be interpreted with caution, however, because sufficient follow-up has not been done of the people reporting these experiences to know whether eventually they will be diagnosed with full-blown schizophrenia or another serious psychiatric disturbance.

Many psychiatrists who treat patients with schizophrenia, if they question the patients specifically, find that they frequently admit to having heard voices as far back as they can remember in childhood and never thought to mention these experiences, as they were perceived as "normal."

Having auditory hallucinations alone certainly does not mean you have, or will have, schizophrenia.

Having auditory hallucinations alone certainly does not mean you have, or will have, schizophrenia. Many people never have any medical or psychiatric problems relating to the voices heard but have them particularly related to falling asleep or just waking (not being fully alert).

Another difference has to do with the nature of the voices. Hearing someone calling your name or sounds that do not involve complex language is less serious. The hallmarks of classical schizophrenia are hearing more than one voice conversing with each other about the hearer and/or at least one voice commenting on the hearer's actions. There are also **command hallucinations**, giving the hearer orders to carry out some action. These latter experiences are certainly more disturbing and characteristic of illness. They rarely, however, stand alone and are accompanied by either some form of bizarre behavior or multiple delusions.

Command hallucinations

Imaginary voices that tell the hearer what to do.

9. What is catatonia?

Catatonic behavior is the extreme of being disorganized and can either be complete immobility and muteness or, at the opposite end, extreme disorganized excitability—an extreme frenzy-like behavior. In its moderate form, it is less extreme, but characterized by a syndrome of repetitive motor movements and frequently failure to speak when talked to. The extreme form of **catatonia** in its full-blown syndrome is actually rare today in the United States and Western nations, although it can be seen more frequently in impoverished countries where patients do not get ample care and the newest pharmaceutical treatments available. Patients with classical catatonia are often quite remarkable in their appearance. They have what has

Catatonia

A condition that is characterized by extremes in behavior, of which the individual appears to be unaware. These behaviors include being mute or in a stupor and immobile, or, at the other extreme, being in an excitatory state of extreme frenzy or agitated excitement.

been termed "waxy flexibility." That is, they stand in one position with their limbs stationary until a person moves them to another position, where they will stay until again moved by another person. A currently practicing young U.S. psychiatrist may never have seen such cases.

Nevertheless, one patient I remember clearly from the mid-1980s (when catatonia was already rare) was a young man who had driven himself to the outpatient clinic. After approaching the check-in desk, however, the receptionist looked up to find him immobile, stiff, and mute. I led him to a private room. He responded several minutes later, but only after having been administered a **tranquilizer** intramuscularly. He denied that anything unusual was happening and was aware that we were discussing him, but he had no explanation for why he had not responded. He then drove home without incident but frequently reentered my office in that same manner.

Tranquilizer

Any drug that is used to calm or pacify an anxious and/or agitated person. There are minor and major classes of tranquilizers that have different chemical properties and are indicated for different psychiatric conditions. The minor ones are for anxiety in a person who has not lost a sense of reality but who needs calming. Major tranquilizers are the class of drugs used for psychotic symptoms.

I also recall a memorable experience when visiting the National Psychiatric Hospital in El Salvador in early 2001. Touring this hospital that was so ill equipped compared with U.S. public psychiatric hospitals was a startling awakening to the status of current psychiatric care in impoverished developing countries. High doses of old medicines were used, as psychiatrists did not know that newer drugs existed, nor did they have them available for use. The floors of the wards had drains to collect the urine that often was uncontrollably produced. What mainly stood out, however, were the several immobile individuals with classical catatonic schizophrenia exhibiting pronounced waxy flexibility. Unfortunately, we do not understand the biologic mechanism that underlies this condition, and because it has become so rare over recent years, it is understudied. In general it is thought today that catatonia usually does not respond to antipsychotic drugs, but rather to the anxiolytic agents, such as clonazepam. Nevertheless, I also had such a patient whose catatonic symptoms responded well to the atypical antipsychotic, Clozapine.

10. What is the course of the illness over time?

No clear predictors of illness course exist, and hopefully, in the future, more biologic variables will be affirmed. Females tend to have a milder course of illness and a later age of onset than males by a mean of about 2 years. Early age of onset and poor premorbid social and academic functioning are hallmarks of a more severe course of illness. The old adage, however, is that one-third of first-episode cases of schizophrenia go on to a chronic deteriorating course. One-third are in the middle with illness but can function (albeit at a lower level than previously), and one-third never have another episode again. The latter statistic is now thought to be overly optimistic. Although many individuals do quite well, particularly if they are treated early and have good family support, continual medication is the key. It is now believed that no more than 10% of individuals who have a clear first episode of schizophrenia can consider themselves recovered afterward without medication. Many additional people may find that they essentially have no symptoms while on medication. Others may be recovered, only to relapse again as long as 5 years later.

Unfortunately, many patients after recovery from the acute stages of a first episode, think that they do not need medication, stop taking it, and eventually relapse. Additionally, the time to a second episode varies. Often it does not occur immediately but may take a few years to again develop. Currently, with the advent of new medications that have almost no side effects, a stable dose can be achieved for a period of several years without the patient feeling the uncomfortable side effects of the old medications. The course of illness in the population as a whole may have changed and become milder as a result of early vigorous treatment with new medications and better compliance among patients. If left untreated, the natural course of schizophrenia is a lifetime of symptoms and deterioration.

If left untreated, the natural course of schizophrenia is a lifetime of symptoms and deterioration.

Before the widespread use of neuroleptic medications, patients were hospitalized for years and lived the rest of their lives on the "back wards" of public hospitals, deteriorating in behavior and **cognition**. It was hard to distinguish between this course of illness and the environmentally deprived effects of institutionalization. When government legislation for the establishment of community mental health centers became in vogue in the 1960s to 1970s, medicated patients were discharged from hospitals and returned to the community. The effects of long-term institutionalization were recognized, but not solved. Often the living environments that patients were transferred to were in many ways impoverished and unsupportive to the needs of these individuals. As a consequence of this dreary and problematic environment and partially the underlying illness itself, many patients returned frequently to the hospitals, and the so-called revolving door phenomenon began to take effect. Throughout their lifetime, patients began to have records filled with numerous admissions and discharges. State-allotted funds for the inpatient institutions have dwindled each year, resulting in the maximum number of beds per state hospital being only a few hundred, or even none in those hospitals that have closed. It is common to drive now through the grounds of the state facilities—once lively,

Cognition

The quality of the mind that allows animals to think, reason, and manipulate their environment to survive. Cognition can be measured by psychological tests.

self-sustaining communities in themselves—and see many buildings boarded up and vacant and weeds growing widely on the surrounding, once patient-manicured, grounds. As evidenced by such closures, one would be led to believe that serious mental illness is disappearing, but this is actually untrue. The incidence and prevalence of schizophrenia worldwide is the same as it has been for decades. Thus, what has changed is that the political mandate has been to close the psychiatric hospitals and to limit the number of inpatient beds that are available. Thus, unless the community is well-equipped with properly-staffed foster homes to care for these individuals, they are emptied out onto the streets often despite the need for a structured inpatient caring environmental setting and become the problem of the cities themselves. Nevertheless, what has also changed is that we are attenuating the course of illness with new medications so that more patients are able to be cared for directly in the community.

Currently, mental health care is in a crisis in the United States (as is health care in general). With serious mental illness, this is an international crisis, of the proportion of the AIDS or other infectious disease epidemics. Schizophrenia is a lifetime disorder that can now be effectively treated and cared for, but legislation needs to be in place that is sensitive to the needs of the disabled individuals with this disease instead of stigmatizing them and thus ignoring their need for care as a result. Nevertheless, the aforementioned history of care for the mentally ill in the United States and other westernized countries hopefully is part of the past. There is current optimism that if continually medicated, people with schizophrenia now can lead normal productive lives without being burdened by uncomfortable symptoms or medication side effects.

11. What exactly is considered a delusion?

A delusion is defined as a fixed false belief that remains despite evidence to the contrary. Many times it is difficult to distinguish "real" delusions from cultural norms or outside stresses that are happening to individuals. For example, I once had a patient who worked as a secretary for the CIA. She claimed that her phone was "bugged" and people were following her. Was this a delusion or could it have been happening because of the nature of her job?

Besides paranoid delusions, there are many classical ones that patients with schizophrenia often describe, including:

- Believing that the commentators on the TV are talking directly to them
- Feeling that they are on a stage and everyone is acting as if this is not real life
- Thinking that people can hear their thoughts or that their thoughts are on a loudspeaker, as if broadcast
- Thinking that their thoughts are not their own and someone else has inserted them into their minds, or even that someone has taken their own thoughts out
- Believing that an external force is controlling their movements and actions.

Other frequent delusions described by patients include believing that their dental fillings have transmitters attached that control their mind or thinking that someone has implanted metal into their body that transmits radio waves. Sometimes the delusions are considered grandiose, such as believing themselves to be a movie star or to have a special mission that God has requested. Delusions can also be even more bizarre, such as having a theory that is completely fiction about the origins and working of the universe or of how the brain works.

With respect to religious beliefs, sometimes it is particularly difficult to separate excessive religiosity from delusionary experiences. For example, as a young psychiatrist, I worked not far from a revival church in which congregations would assemble and sing progressively louder until members were drawn into chanting trances, almost as if they had no control over their actions. They were so overcome by the event that one could perceive them to be in acute psychotic states. When the music stopped and the meeting was over, however, each individual returned to an ordinary state. When religious beliefs and a preoccupation with these beliefs interfere with one's social and daily life and occupational and educational achievements, you can call the beliefs a "symptom" of a disorder. Certainly this is one illustration that psychopathology is likely to be on a continuum in many ways between what is considered normal by society and what is considered abnormal by psychiatrists.

Debates exist about whether schizophrenia actually exists other than in the imagination of psychiatrists. Although this view is certainly extreme, the cultural environment of a newly presenting patient needs to be considered before a diagnosis is made. The disorder that is described in this book is more than extreme views that can be related to culture. It affects individuals from all cultural backgrounds and races equally, and many of the delusions are more similar than they are different across cultures. How you separate "beliefs" that have no scientific proof from "delusions" that can be defined as pathological is a matter of philosophical debate that will undoubtedly continue over time. It is, however, beyond the scope of this book.

12. What is meant by "positive" and "negative" symptoms?

Positive symptoms are those that produce activity. They include things that are said, acted on, or clearly disturb the individual, such as delusions and hallucinations. **Negative symptoms** (the so-called defect state) are things that are lacking in activity or reduce it—thus "negative." They include a lack of movement, speech, emotional expression, social ability, or initiative to do anything. Positive symptoms tend to fluctuate and respond better to current medications than negative symptoms. Negative symptoms are more stable over time and may be present in the beginning of the illness but are more manifest when the illness becomes chronic and can be the only signs of illness in the stabilized "residual" cases. It is thought that the newer **"atypical" antipsychotic medications**, such as clozapine, olanzapine, quetiapine, risperidone, and others, may have an effect on reducing negative symptoms. Sometimes depressive symptoms can overlap with negative ones. Since patients with schizophrenia can benefit from antidepressant medication for episodes of depression, these must also be carefully distinguished.

Positive symptoms

Considered the active symptoms of hallucinations and delusions of schizophrenia.

Negative symptoms

Those characteristics of psychiatric illness that present as withdrawn behavior, an expressionless face, a lack of initiative, a lack of interest, slow speech, slowed thoughts, and slowed movements.

Atypical antipsychotic medications

These are newer medications that were first developed by drug companies in the 1990s for use in schizophrenia and are sometimes also called the second generation of drugs. Because they have different biochemical effects in the brain compared to the older drugs, such as Thorazine or Haldol, and thus are less likely to cause the typical motor disturbances seen with these drugs, they have been called "atypical."

13. Do people with schizophrenia have language problems?

Frequently, a patient with schizophrenia in an acute state may speak in a very disorganized and loose manner whereby sentences don't appear to be connected by logical meaning. For example, a typical utterance might be, "I just saw a man walk down the street to open the door. But why is he throwing the ball? Do you know where the soda bottle came from? Doctor, can you get me out of this jail?" And so on. However, patients with schizophrenia do not always speak in such obviously mixed-up fashion; they may instead have more subtle peculiarities of language that can be detected only by psychological testing.

Regardless of whether obvious language deficits are present, the major symptoms of schizophrenia can all be explained by an underlying disorder in the brain pathways that process language, both that which is perceived and that which is spoken. For example, if the brain perceives people speaking in an abnormal way so that the connections between the auditory center and the center for meanings in the brain are abnormal, then the hearer will think that something unreal has been said; delusions are then the manifestation. The patient has thus put an erroneous meaning onto what someone has said. If, on the other hand, an individual is having reflective thoughts about himself or herself but the auditory pathways are misconnected in the brain region that distinguishes what is heard from what is thought, then the thoughts might appear to be actually heard from outside of one's head.

The disorganization of language can more directly be seen as a symptom of these misconnections and can occur in the more severe cases. The negative symptoms of schizophrenia may be either directly caused by language pathway deficits, such as in a lack of complex speech or in a lack of content of speech, or by a secondary result of the positive symptoms that are disturbing and preoccupying. Much debate has existed about the relationship of all these symptoms to the primary cause of the illness, but little progress toward a better understanding of the illness has come out of these discussions.

Studies of children who later developed schizophrenia are interesting because some have been shown to have had a delay in the development of language such that the pre-schizophrenic individual will say his or her first words later than most children and put them into sentences even later. Learning to read is also delayed in these children to a varying degree. This slowing of the acquisition of the building blocks for language suggests abnormalities in the timing and construction of brain pathways for language.

14. Do people with schizophrenia get depression?

Depression is more commonly a characteristic symptom of schizophrenia than most clinicians have realized. In fact, the majority of patients with chronic schizophrenia have had an episode of major depression at some time in the course of their illness. Often the first onset of schizophrenia will be preceded by several months of what patients will describe as a depression. In addition, as an episode of acute schizophrenia resolves, depression may follow. Sometimes, however, depressive symptoms can be confused with negative symptoms of slowed and decreased speech, slowed movements, a lack of interest in activities, and general withdrawal. It is when depression can predominate over psychotic symptoms that the diagnosis of schizoaffective disorder or even bipolar disorder might be considered.

Often the first onset of schizophrenia will be preceded by several months of what patients will describe as a depression.

Alzheimer's disease

One of a few progressive brain diseases that has been more frequently diagnosed recently in older people who appear disoriented and have difficulty communicating properly with others.

15. Are memory problems symptoms of schizophrenia?

Schizophrenia is clearly distinguishable from **Alzheimer's disease**, where recent memory problems are the hallmark. A subtle cognitive disturbance, however, is also clearly present in patients with schizophrenia and at an early stage of illness. It is now known from some large research studies that IQ falls somewhat just before the onset of illness and particularly that verbal memory and measures of what is called short-term **working memory** are often impaired throughout the illness. However, most studies fail to find that these deficits in

Working memory

A contemporary term for short-term memory. It is thought of as an active system for temporarily storing and manipulating information needed for conducting complex tasks such as learning, reasoning, and comprehending things.

cognition are progressive after the start of a full-blown illness, which may be because the greatest change in cognitive functioning and abilities seems to occur during a prodromal stage of the illness—i.e., in that period when changes are occurring over a 1- to 2-year period before the person with schizophrenia is noticed to be ill by those around him or her. Some of the cognitive changes may also stem from an early brain or adolescent developmental problem. The prodromal stage of schizophrenia varies considerably in length; some patients never appear normal from early childhood, while others do well until late adolescence and have a more sudden abrupt downhill course in functioning.

The underlying cause of the impairments and their mechanisms are not known. For example, is there a memory information retrieval problem, as some studies seem to suggest, or is there an information storage problem? Sometimes the memory and learning problems are confused with an attention problem. Regardless, people with schizophrenia do not learn new things, particularly of a complex sequential nature, as well as do people without schizophrenia. It is assumed that the cognitive problems stem from structural and thus functional brain disturbances in the frontal and temporal cortices of the brain, particularly on the left side, regions where language is processed.

Some medications, such as Cogentin, used to treat the side effects of some of the older neuroleptic medications, can have an effect on memory, and this should be taken into account during evaluations of memory problems.

16. Do people with schizophrenia have a low IQ?

Most individuals with schizophrenia have normal intelligence; however, there is a drop in each individual's IQ at the beginning of illness. Some studies show that individuals with high IQs have a better overall outcome of a schizophrenic episode than people with lower IQs and thus are somewhat protected. In contrast, however, some mental retardation syndromes do co-occur with schizophrenia and, when present, may give clues to the origin of the disorder in those individuals. Usually these cases have very poor premorbid histories, the individuals having been educated in special classes in childhood and administered many treatments before adolescence.

17. Are muscular problems associated with schizophrenia?

It used to be thought that any motor problems present in people with schizophrenia, such as the well-known severe example of tardive **dyskinesia**, were a consequence of medications. It is now recognized, and was many decades ago, that some motor disturbance and strange movements known as dyskinesias are present in patients as they are becoming ill and before they took any medications. In fact, some studies show that motor development is somewhat delayed during early childhood in people who later develop schizophrenia (e.g., age at first walking), and even at birth some abnormal clumsy movements were detected by one investigator (Elaine Walker, Atlanta) in some now-famous home movies.

Dyskinesia

Difficulty in performing movements voluntarily.

18. Do people with schizophrenia have a reduced life span or die from their illness?

It is doubtful that schizophrenia directly reduces the life span. There are even debates as to whether incidences of certain cancers are rarer among people with schizophrenia than in the general population. If large populations are studied, however, the age at death is lower in people with schizophrenia because of proneness to accidents, increased suicide rates, chronic institutionalization in the past that may have led to a lack of rigorous health care and proper nutrition, as well as acceleration of aging because of the multiple combinations of medications with many adverse side effects that people with chronic schizophrenia tend to be taking for many years. Still, today people with schizophrenia tend not to obtain the adequate health care and preventive dietary and health-related measures that can work toward increasing one's life span. This is a public health problem that needs to be addressed. There have not been enough research studies examining the ways in which people with schizophrenia go through the aging process.

19. Are there medical conditions that look like schizophrenia?

Countless other illnesses are sometimes accompanied by hallucinations and delusions, from metabolic disturbances influencing the brain to viral illnesses, brain tumors, and specific chromosomal abnormalities. The specific aspect of the auditory hallucinations, however, might be different. For example, more than one voice talking about the individual or one voice commenting on the individual's actions is more specific to schizophrenia. The course of illness is more characteristic as well, and can be an indication. All the other mentioned causes have other physical symptoms accompanying the psychosis that are uncharacteristic of schizophrenia. When someone presents to a physician with what appears to be a first episode of schizophrenia, good medical practice indicates that these other conditions should be excluded, particularly if there is any indication that they might be present or the characteristics that are seen on the first episode are in any way atypical. Some of the examples, both common and rare, of medical illnesses that can mask as schizophrenia are phenylketonuria, Huntington's Chorea, lupus erythematosus, thyroid disease, parathyroid disease, brain tumors, viral encephalitis, and chronic alcohol and drug abuse. These are just a few examples of many.

20. Do people with schizophrenia have fewer offspring?

Fertility and **fecundity** are two different entities. People with schizophrenia, if withdrawn and behaviorally different, may not want mates and may not appear attractive to others. Their difficulties in forming close relations generalize to sexual problems as well. This is truer of males than of females, as evidenced by some studies, which show that males with schizophrenia have fewer offspring than do females. This reduced number of offspring is thought to be, thus, a fecundity problem and is not likely caused by reduced fertility for biologic reasons. Still, it is possible that some causes of schizophrenia, such as chromosomal microdeletions and chromosomal insertions, could as a tertiary effect lead to reduced fertility. Thus, one may wonder, why is an illness that leads to reduced offspring not decreasing?

Fertility

Having the normal biology that gives one the ability to bear children.

Fecundity

Bearing children.

Although in some diseases that continue despite reduced or nonexistent fertility a genetic advantage is associated with the disadvantageous illness (such as in the case of sickle cell anemia and protection from malaria), no such relationship has been described for schizophrenia. Why schizophrenia still exists today, given its genetic tendency, and is not declining in incidence is still unclear and a curious question for researchers to explore.

21. Are there some societies in which no individuals develop schizophrenia?

This is a hotly debated issue. E. Fuller Torrey (1980), in his book *Schizophrenia and Civilization*, described clusters of schizophrenia throughout the world and some isolated areas where it is nonexistent. He particularly described the highlands of Papua New Guinea as one region without evidence of schizophrenia. Currently, however, psychiatrists practicing in Papua New Guinea say that Torrey certainly missed some cases, and documents of such cases do exist in the literature. It would be interesting to study these societies closer. For example, the San tribe of South Africa is said to be the oldest African group in existence; it has isolated itself from society, maintaining its prehistoric hunter–gatherer culture despite the surrounding civilization. Although there is some indication that schizophrenia does exist among these people, because of tribal laws, it has been difficult for Western-trained professionals to enter their communities to examine whether mental illness exists within the context of their culture.

Despite these rare examples, the World Health Organization has conducted studies over the years to show that schizophrenia is a disease of humanity and is universal. This fact alone may give clues to its genetic origin. A new gene mutation would be very unlikely to cause schizophrenia, as modern **Homo sapiens** were derived from one bottleneck formed in Africa approximately 150,000 years ago. For a genetic disorder to be universal, it must be as old as modern humans themselves. Since the capacity for complex language is distinctly human and schizophrenia can be seen as a disorder of the biologic pathways for language, a **gene** or genes that define the capacity for language may somehow be related to schizophrenia (Crow, 1997; DeLisi, 2001). Alternatively, the hypothesis that multiple rare spontaneous mutations—perhaps in specific genes that have a tendency for this to occur, could be the genetic mechanism involved and the reason why schizophrenia does not die out despite reduced fecundity.

Homo sapiens

The scientific designation for modern human beings.

Gene

A functional unit of heredity that is in a fixed place in the structure of a chromosome.

PART TWO

Treatment: When, Where, by Whom, and with What?

What type of professional can treat the first symptoms of schizophrenia?

Do I have to be treated in a hospital if I have schizophrenia, and if so, for how long?

What are the current choices for medication?

More . . .

"In the midst of this godless kneeling, I suddenly remembered that I had forgotten to take my lithium. . . . I reached into my purse for my medication, opened the bottle and immediately dropped all of the pills onto the cathedral floor. The floor was filthy, there were people all around, and I was too embarrassed to bend over and pick up the pills."

—Kay Redfield Jamison on a trip to Canterbury Cathedral from her autobiographical revelations about her bouts with psychiatric illness in *An Unquiet Mind,* 1995

22. What type of professional can treat the first symptoms of schizophrenia?

Many types of doctors and therapists are currently treating the first symptoms of schizophrenia, and because of the types of health services in the United States and other similar countries, the general practitioner, family physician, pediatrician, or emergency room doctor will likely be the first to identify the symptoms. Since the early warning signs can sometimes be indistinguishable from adolescent mood changes, general practitioners and pediatricians will often suggest that the patients will "grow out of it" and that parental controls are necessary. Many cases have been made public of severely disturbed adolescents whose families and healthcare professionals, initially aware of their behavior, did not understand that an impending psychosis could be approaching. The Columbine High School murders in Colorado were certainly an example. The parents and teachers seemed largely unaware that delusional and bizarre changes were taking place in the boys who had paired together out of common extreme thoughts and interests. They were saying things and acting in a manner that those around them should have been able to detect as serious pathology that was brewing. Instead, they had been in a juvenile detention program and actually had social workers who did not notice their downward spiraling.

Several similar school incidences have since been reported in the news. The lack of proper identification of those first symptoms before they become a devastating crisis and harmful to other people or themselves is common. Another famous occurrence, the "Long Island Railroad Massacre," was caused by a young adult who for several months became increasingly paranoid and delusional, but his symptoms remained unrecognized by all around him until he boarded a commuter train one evening from Penn Station, New York, with a rifle and shot several passengers randomly. Although cases do not all culminate in a violent act before being recognized, these are extreme examples of what can happen when subtle signs are ignored by even people close to the person who is becoming ill.

Although general nonpsychiatric doctors may end up treating people with early schizophrenia, the best treatment will certainly be from trained psychiatrists who are versed in the early signs and latest medications, their doses, efficacy, and side effects and when and how long to medicate. In addition, specifically trained psychiatrists are knowledgeable about providing the needed follow-up and long-term care. This type of care is of course the ideal situation, recognizing that many people with schizophrenia in the United States may quickly use up their health insurance benefits or not be covered at all. The medications are expensive, as is the continued care, and people with schizophrenia tend not to obtain high-paying employment or maintain regular jobs with benefits. In fact, during the prodromal stage, which often lasts a couple of years, it is not uncommon for an individual to lose a job or drop out of college and thus forfeit insurance benefits.

23. Does a psychiatrist always need to be seen and how frequently?

Pharmacotherapy

Treatment of disease through the use of drugs.

Cognitive behavioral therapy (CBT)

A brief form of treatment based on the principle that the way one thinks about something causes actions. Thus, it is focused on changing thinking patterns that lead to disruptive behavior.

Although general practitioners, psychologists, nurse practitioners, and social workers who all practice psychotherapy may deal with patients with schizophrenia in their practice, psychiatrists (as stated previously) know how to use the latest treatments. **Pharmacotherapy** is the primary treatment modality and is prescribed only through a medical doctor or licensed nurse practitioner. Although other therapies given by social workers or psychologists can help, such as supportive psychotherapy, **cognitive behavioral therapy (CBT)**, family therapy, and orthomolecular therapy (vitamin and mineral treatments), *only* pharmacotherapy will relieve the symptoms. The others are only supplements to medication and may facilitate and augment their effects, but do not replace them. The non-pharmacotherapies may also help in daily functioning in a way that medication alone cannot. Pharmacotherapy certainly does not have all the answers; for example, some patients do not respond well to medications and may even have uncomfortable side effects. Medications do not yet "cure" the actual biologic basis for the illness but are likely to be effective for suppressing the symptoms, much like aspirin suppresses the fever and headache from influenza.

After a patient is stabilized on medication, the psychotherapist, social workers, and occupational therapists need to take a role in providing the social treatments that are needed to improve the quality of life of people with schizophrenia. Rarely will a psychiatrist, who has many patients on his or her rolls, have or take the time to follow up on a patient's practical needs or to make sure that the patient complies with the proper medication regime and other services. The role of other professionals is essential for the support necessary to achieve a favorable outcome for the illness of each patient.

24. Why do some psychiatrists not treat people with schizophrenia?

The average clinical psychiatrist rarely treats people with schizophrenia, at least in the United States, for several reasons. The first is that doctors fear liability from lawsuits if the patient does something harmful to himself or herself or to others. These clinicians also fear the violence and aggression toward themselves when they frequently practice in isolated private office settings. The second reason is that people with schizophrenia have limited resources and are almost always unemployed on a regular basis. The nature of their illness means that they will have difficulty working and have no insurance coverage. Even when patients come from families with considerable financial security, they can quickly drain parental savings. Psychiatrists in private practice can rarely see patients with schizophrenia and maintain a livelihood. Thus, these patients are generally seen in clinics by physicians/psychiatrists who have large caseloads and are then followed up by caseworkers and psychiatric social workers. Unfortunately, many people with schizophrenia never make it into a stable treatment setting and are lost to follow-up either after hospitalizations for acute episodes or because they leave the security of a parental home with support and wander away aimlessly, sometimes living on the street as a result of the symptoms.

People with schizophrenia have limited resources and are almost always unemployed on a regular basis.

25. What if I do not have insurance or if my policy does not cover psychiatric care?

Although a lack of insurance is clearly a serious problem with health care today in America and some other countries, the current system is not hopeless. Some public hospital emergency rooms will provide acute care and then make referrals to the appropriate clinic. The social worker assigned to the emergency room often knows what is available in your area and also funds that can be applied for to help in individual situations. In addition, there are sliding pay scales and many kind-hearted psychiatrists who will not allow the patient to pay more than he or she can afford, although admittedly these people are far too few.

The U.S. federal government has recently passed legislation for "parity in health care" for mental illness. Congress must recognize that schizophrenia and other psychiatric disorders are medical illnesses that warrant coverage that is equal to diabetes, hypertension, and other chronic illnesses. This has taken a lot of public education, and it has been difficult to get Congress to bring such a bill onto the floor of the House and Senate. Congress deferred the effective date of the *Mental Health Parity and Addiction Equity Act of 2008* sponsored by Senators Paul Wellstone and Pete Domenici to January 2010 for plans that otherwise would have been covered in 2009. The Mental Health Parity and Addiction Equity Act amends the Employee Retirement Income Security Act and the Public Health Service Act to prohibit employers' health plans from imposing any caps or limitations on mental health treatment or substance use disorder benefits that are not applied to medical and surgical benefits. The Mental Health Parity and Addiction Equity Act does not require health insurance plans to provide mental health or substance use disorder benefits. However, for group health plans with 50 or more employees that choose to provide mental health and substance use disorder benefits, the Act does require parity with medical and surgical benefits.

Thus, group health plans that provide both medical and surgical benefits and mental health and substance use disorder benefits may not impose financial requirements and treatment limitations applicable to mental health and substance use disorder benefits that are more restrictive than the financial requirements and treatment limitations applied to medical and surgical benefits. Requirements such as co-payments and deductibles and limitations such as number of visits or frequency of treatments can be no more restrictive on mental health and substance use disorder benefits than the requirements or limitations imposed on medical and surgical benefits.

Another way to find appropriate healthcare services is to find the nearest National Alliance on Mental Illness (NAMI) chapter. NAMI will have knowledge of the best places to go for immediate treatment and will be able to give advice based on experience often with their own family members. They serve not only as a resource in difficult times but as important continued support for people dealing with mental illness in their families.

26. Do I have to be treated in a hospital if I have schizophrenia, and, if so, for how long?

Often, unfortunately, the first time patients' symptoms of schizophrenia are noticed is when they are psychotic (no awareness of reality to the point that they could be harmful to themselves or others). In this case, patients rarely volunteer to go to a hospital and are either forcefully brought there by family or friends, or picked up by the police.

In many countries, particularly in impoverished nations, the progress in modernizing hospitals is far behind the Western world, and the reputation of psychiatric hospitals is such that after someone is placed there, he or she is thought to disappear and not come back. There is thus a terrible fear of psychiatric "institutions." Often the hospitals are so ill equipped and ill staffed that they become more a way to isolate people from society than a facility for humanely treating patients with the latest medications. For example, such was the case when I visited the National Psychiatric Hospital in El Salvador. It surprised me that even the library where psychiatrists should be able to get the latest advice was void of major journals. Only outdated copies of *The American Journal of Psychiatry* from 10 years ago were on the shelves. In other countries, such as within central Africa, relatives keep afflicted individuals chained to walls or doorknobs of homes in order to keep them from harming themselves or other people. Much publicity occurred many years ago about the conditions of psychiatric hospitals in America, becoming material for Hollywood movies such as *The Snake Pit* that I viewed as a child or *One Flew Over the Cuckoo's Nest* from the 1970s. Even most recently the movie *Changeling* with Angelina Jolie provokes images of psychiatric hospitals that have long been forgotten, at least in the United States.

Truthfully, many years ago lobotomies were practiced as *One Flew Over the Cuckoo's Nest* depicts, and patients lived in squalor as in *The Snake Pit*. Times, however, have clearly changed. Most general hospitals in the United States and other industrialized nations have psychiatry wards, and patients with schizophrenia are kept only as long as required to be stabilized on medication and get into proper longer term outpatient treatment (usually 10 to 30 days). Often hospitalization is best for the patient once medications are started because not only can the patient be under close observation for side effects, but also it takes time for the medications to work, and during that period, the illness could escalate.

27. What treatments were used before pharmaceutical companies introduced neuroleptic medication?

The history of treatment for schizophrenia is interesting and is available in several very readable books, although many espouse the authors' prejudices against psychiatry more than relay the facts (Fink, 1999; Whitaker, 2002). A recent best-selling novel in the United Kingdom, *Human Traces* (by Sebastian Faulks) gives an interesting historical account of the treatment of people with mental illness over a century ago; but unfortunately this book strays somewhat from historical truth when it endows its psychiatrists with the creative hypothesis about the uniquely human nature of schizophrenia that was actually formulated a century later (Crow, 1997).

People with the symptoms of schizophrenia have always stood out in society as not belonging because of the extreme oddness in the way they look or act. Thus, they have often been dubbed "crazy," "loco," "mad," and so on. During the late 1800s to the early twentieth century and even before, there was a big movement in America and Europe to create large psychiatric institutions to house these individuals and place them far from urban areas. This focus on the question of management of the mentally ill led some to believe that schizophrenia was actually increasing in epidemic proportions throughout Western civilization (Torrey and Miller, 2000), although most researchers believe that this illusion has no scientific basis but rather is due to changes in diagnostic systems and definitions of **insanity** and the different psychotic conditions.

Insanity
Unsoundness of mind, characterized by lack of rational judgment so that the individual cannot manage his affairs or conform to social standards and thus understand what is morally right or wrong. This term is also used in criminal law, to find someone "not guilty by reason of insanity."

Much of the treatment during these times was primarily isolation from society. Various therapies were given, however, including restraints (such as chaining), packing in ice, bloodletting, and even tooth removal. Through a great part of the twentieth century, most hospital wards had not only baths for placing people in cold-packs, but also isolation rooms on every ward so that agitated patients could be taken away from the rest of the patients and staff. While the latter are still important parts of psychiatric wards today, their use is restricted and well monitored. Many years ago, patients were frequently in these rooms for longer than necessary because of the staff's fear. On some rare occasions, patients who may have been misdiagnosed and were withdrawing from addictive drugs or had cardiac problems unfortunately died while in this kind of therapy. Insulin shock therapy was a popular treatment. One drug, a forerunner of the neuroleptics, was reserpine, which was used frequently until phenothiazines became widespread. In addition, by the mid-twentieth century, psychoanalysis for schizophrenia became popular and was practiced well into the 1970s in some famous institutions for the well-to-do—notably, the Menninger Clinic in Kansas and Chestnut Lodge in Maryland. Chestnut Lodge, a beautifully situated campus with lavish rooms and dining facilities and a lovely swimming pool for patient exercise, exposed people to the therapies developed by the well-known analyst Frieda-Fromm Reichmann and became popularized by the novel *I Never Promised You a Rose Garden*. Patients were said to need psychoanalytic regression back to infancy and then mothering again through the stages of development, slowly for symptomatic improvement and regaining a proper sense of reality. In the 1980s, Chestnut Lodge was threatened with losing its accreditation unless neuroleptics were reinstated in the treatment regime for all patients with schizophrenia, and thus, the institution gradually lost the attraction it once had for wealthy families of affected individuals. It eventually closed as a mental hospital in 2001 due to financial problems and was bought by a national health corporation to house medical treatments, then later turned into a school, and currently condominiums. In June of 2009 the historic main building of the hospital, which appeared in movies, was destroyed by fire.

In the early part of the twentieth century, Egas Moniz in Portugal developed a new technique (for which he received the Nobel Prize in Medicine) called *leukotomy*. This surgical procedure involved drilling holes in the skull above the temporal lobes and then with the use of a needle-like instrument disrupting connections in brain tissue from several regions of the frontal lobes. This procedure was reported to alleviate the anxiety, agitation, and uncontrollable psychological stress of severely ill institutionalized mental patients. Shortly afterward, Walter J. Freeman adopted this technique in the United States and performed a few thousand leukotomies (renamed **lobotomy**) in many patients during the peak of its popularity in the mid-1900s (El-Hai, 2005).

Lobotomy

The surgical division of one or more brain tracts. It is usually referred to as cutting nerves that run from the frontal lobe to the thalamus in the brain. It has been done in various ways, most often by inserting a needle above the nose in between the eyes. It is also known as leukotomy.

From the late 1930s through the 1950s, lobotomies were widely accepted as good practice in psychiatry throughout the mental hospitals in the United States. Although some individuals were dramatically helped by this procedure, there was also much abuse of its use, extending the indications for lobotomies to patients who the nursing staff simply found "difficult" and behavioral problems in the social setting of institutional life. Even the very wealthy and well-connected families (as in the famous case of Rosemary Kennedy) had lobotomies performed unscrupulously on affected

There are still some parts of the world, such as countries of South America, where lobotomies are currently being performed, although this practice has long been discontinued in the United States and most Westernized countries.

family members. There are still some parts of the world, such as countries of South America, where lobotomies are currently being performed, although this practice has long been discontinued in the United States and most Westernized countries.

28. What are the current choices for medication?

Antipsychotic

Any medication that specifically suppresses the positive symptoms of hallucinations and delusions. This medication can also be useful in other conditions as a strong tranquilizer.

Since the 1960s, **antipsychotic** medication has been the mainstay treatment for schizophrenia, and the outcome is better if individuals with schizophrenia receive this treatment early in the course of the illness. In fact, it has been said that the new medications "emptied" the psychiatric hospitals of the long-term patients in the 1960s and brought people with schizophrenia into the mainstream of society. Severe variable side effects of these medications still existed, however, and doses went higher and higher to achieve clinical effect. Many patients still did not respond even to very high doses.

The prototype of all these drugs was Thorazine, a phenothiazine. There were many drugs of this class introduced by different companies in those days, and while they had the same overall effects on suppressing the positive symptoms of schizophrenia, their side effects varied, with different relative chances with each for sedation, producing hypotension, tremors and stiffness, and lowering the seizure threshold (these were Thorazine, Trilafon, Stelazine, Prolixin). Shortly afterwards, drugs with similar clinical and receptor profiles (but different chemical structures) were developed (e.g., Moban, Navane, Haldol). All these first-generation drugs were thought to exert their action predominantly by blocking one of the dopamine receptors (labeled D_2) but had other receptor actions as well and were not considered "clean drugs" chemically.

In the 1970s, clozapine was introduced in Europe and had remarkable effects in patients who did not respond to the usual medications. This drug was thought to have a greater effect on serotonin receptors and thus a very different receptor profile than the first-generation drugs. However, when cases were reported of life-threatening leukopenia caused by clozapine, and in rare instances when some patients died, its use was limited and its placement on the market in the United States was delayed. By the late 1980s, however, there was renewed interest in clozapine in the United States, and reports were making the newspapers of miraculous recoveries of individuals who were completely psychotic and thought-disordered before clozapine who on the drug had become "normal," were speaking coherently, were well groomed, were able to be released from the hospital, and were applying for employment. New trials were begun in the United States, and the FDA (Food and Drug Administration) then finally approved the use of clozapine for treatment of patients with tardive dyskinesia, as it appeared only very rarely to lead to the reduced white blood cell counts that were highly noted previously in Europe. It was also approved for patients who were nonresponsive to other medications and continues to be a drug that can produce remarkable effects in those who have a severe illness that doesn't completely respond to other drugs. It was later noted that clozapine seemed to have a unique effect on preventing suicidal tendencies. Individuals treated with clozapine, however, have to be closely monitored with blood testing to assure that they did not develop blood dyscrasias, such as the leukopenia seen in the past. Thus, its value today as a primary treatment for schizophrenia should not be overlooked. No cases of serious leukopenia or deaths have been reported since its reinstitution and careful blood monitoring.

In the meantime, many pharmaceutical companies have been developing new drugs for schizophrenia that have similar neurochemical mechanisms, although not identical, to clozapine but that are less toxic to the blood system. Several of these reached the market over the last 2 decades and are available worldwide, although unfortunately less so in the poorer developing countries. These drugs have been dubbed the second-generation neuroleptics, or "atypicals," and include Janssen Pharmaceutica's drug Risperdal (risperidone), Lilly's drug Zyprexa (olanzapine), AstraZeneca's drug Seroquel (quetiapine), Bristol-Myers Squibb's drug Abilify (aripiprazole), and Pfizer's drug Geodon (ziprasidone). These drugs may go by different trade names in other countries, but they are produced by the global offices of all the major companies listed here. Doses and potency vary among these drugs, but in general they have the same efficacy, much lower incidence of side effects, and thus good tolerability compared with the earlier generation of drugs such as Haldol, Thorazine, Mellaril, Trilafon, Navane, and others.

Many chronic patients are still medicated with these first-generation drugs. They are much less expensive, as the drug companies no longer hold patents on them, and their efficacy is really not any different from that of the atypicals, as has been shown in some recent large treatment trials. In addition, in clinical practice, if a patient does not respond to a typical and atypical drug, he or she should be given a trial of clozapine (if this drug has not yet been tried); the incidence of response to clozapine in other-drug nonresponsive patients is still greater than with any of the other drugs. Sometimes in the very difficult and nonresponsive patient, a combination of clozapine and a drug such as Risperdal is helpful, as the synergism between them allows for all the needed receptor blockade to occur, and the Risperdal tends to raise the blood levels of clozapine.

29. Are combinations of different medications more effective than one alone?

Reality is that there appears to be a huge gap between research and clinical practice. Researchers tend to frown on so-called "polypharmacy" and cite in support of their view that there are no good double-blind controlled trials to support polypharmacy. They recommend instead the use of one drug and when it is not effective tapering the patient off that drug and trying another. However, polypharmacy, giving combinations of different drugs having the same actions, appears to be the practice of the great majority of clinical psychiatrists who provide care to chronic patients with schizophrenia. Frequently, patients are found to be administered both typical and atypical neuroleptics combined, with an added mood-stabilizing drug to "calm" them (e.g., valproic acid or carbamazepine). These latter drugs are therapeutic for seizure disorders but also have been used for mania where a patient is agitated and irritable. These drugs appear to take away that edge and thus are called "mood stabilizers." Another such drug that has been useful is lamotrigine. Based on unmet clinical needs and modest evidence from case reports, combinations of two or more second-generation drugs may merit future investigation in efficacy trials involving patients with schizophrenia who have treatment-resistant illness (including partial response) or who are responsive to treatment but develop intolerable adverse effects. Other instances that may merit polypharmacy are when schizophrenia is accompanied by comorbid conditions (e.g., anxiety, suicidal or self-injurious behavior, aggression). In certain clinical situations, antipsychotic cotreatment may be superior to monotherapy. However, the research data thus far are not clear about this practice.

30. What are the medication side effects?

The two side effects of the atypicals that have received a lot of publicity are substantial weight gain, more so with Zyprexa (olanzapine) than with the other drugs, and diabetic-like problems with glucose metabolism. Although each drug company will report studies indicating that their drug has fewer side effects than those of their competitors, and in many areas more efficacy, it is hard to tease out the bias in this reporting. Thus, the National Institute of Mental Health (NIMH) invested funds in a large multicenter comparison trial called CATIE (Clinical Antipsychotic Trials of Intervention Effectiveness) using several of these drugs and one of the older drugs (perphenazine, trade name: Trilafon) as well to compare their efficacy and side effects. Surprisingly, few differences between the drugs have emerged although there was some suggestion that perpehnazine certainly held up against the others and that olanzapine and clozapine had some advantage over the other atypicals for symptom improvement.

The older drugs, such as Haldol, Thorazine, perphenazine (Trilafon), and others, have not been used much in the United States over the past few years because the efficacy of the atypicals has been clearly proven and drug companies tend to push those medications that are still under patent (i.e., the newer atypicals). However, some other countries still predominantly use the older drugs, and thus, motor side effects can still be seen. There is still clearly a role for these drugs in the management of schizophrenia. Mainly, the old medications produced Parkinson-like side effects (tremors and stiffness), and in some cases, tardive dyskinesia was a particularly severe side effect (pronounced uncontrollable motor movements of the limbs and tongue). With the discontinuation of medication, sometimes it was reversible, but often not. Also, trials of discontinuation and then reinstitution of the medications often made tardive dyskinesia even worse. This debilitating condition was widely feared, not only because of the disability it caused but also because of the peculiar look it gave its victims, forcing them to stand out in public and be stigmatized. Other side effects included sedation, dizziness, hypotension, a lack of sexual drive, and hepatic damage.

None of these side effects appears to be a major concern for the newer second-generation antipsychotics, although the metabolic syndrome certainly is. With respect to results of the CATIE study, clozapine was found to be the most efficacious, but for those patients who preferred not to take clozapine, olanzapine and risperidone seemed more effective than ziprasidone and quetiapine. But side effects varied. Olanzapine was associated with substantial weight gain and metabolic problems, more so than the other medications. Ziprasidone (Geodon) was consistently associated with reduction in weight and improvement in metabolic indicators and thus has the least metabolic effects, but does have adverse cardiac side effects that need to be monitored. Risperidone showed the lowest rate of intolerable side effects, but some patients on this drug have had the motor disturbances of the first-generation drugs.

Some words about the metabolic syndrome, which has been the much focused-upon side effect of the newer atypical drugs: The metabolic syndrome is characterized by a group of metabolic risk factors in one person. They include being overweight, particularly with excessive fat tissue around the abdominal region, high blood triglycerides, low-HDL cholesterol, and high-LDL cholesterol. The latter foster fatty deposits in arteries, elevated blood pressure, insulin resistance or glucose intolerance, a prothrombotic state of high fibrinogen or plasminogen activator inhibitor-1 in the blood and also a proinflammatory state with elevated C-reactive protein in the blood. Thus, people with the metabolic syndrome are at increased risk of coronary heart disease and stroke, peripheral vascular disease, and type II diabetes mellitus. Often schizophrenia patients with diabetes tend to have difficulty controlling their blood sugars when they are medicated with drugs such as olanzapine or clozapine.

31. What are the treatments for side effects?

Some medications such as Cogentin and Artane (anticholinergic and antihistaminic) are used solely for treating the tremors and stiffness, but despite these drugs, most patients on the older neuroleptics have had visible effects. There is no effective treatment for tardive dyskinesia. The main treatments for the metabolic syndrome are diet and lowering cholesterol and lipidemia using the new statin class of drugs, as well as controlling lipids in the diet, lowering blood pressure, and controlling diabetes and high blood sugar levels.

32. How long does medication have to be taken?

Treatment is generally long term and is considered necessary for the first decade after symptoms have appeared.

Taking medication for schizophrenia is similar to taking medication for high blood pressure. Although someone who has only one episode of a psychosis should have a closely monitored trial without medications after he or she is free of symptoms for 1 year, in 90% of these cases, the illness does reoccur within the first 5 years. Thus, treatment is generally long term and is considered necessary for the first decade after symptoms have appeared. If some symptoms, even residual negative ones, are still apparent, medication should be taken indefinitely. With recovery, the medication can be slowly tapered after several years and stopped. Not enough research is yet available to determine how long people need to take preventive medication after the symptoms are gone and who will or will not benefit from a lifetime of medications.

33. Are there alternative treatments to medication?

It is generally not believed by psychiatrists that there are alternatives to medications, and the advertisements for so-called alternatives are misleading. There are only supplementary treatments, some of which have no effect, such as vitamins and dietary supplements, and others of which may have some modest effect or have an effect on specific symptoms, such as transcranial magnetic stimulation (TMS). Psychotherapy and family therapy are adjunctive treatments to medication.

34. What is cognitive behavioral therapy?

Cognitive behavioral therapy (CBT) has become a popular treatment for many emotional and behavioral traits. For schizophrenia, it has recently become a popular adjunct to medication at a time when the patient is stabilized but has a baseline of functional disturbances that are not alleviated by medication. In addition, one study in Manchester, England, claims effects on delaying the onset of schizophrenia by treatment with CBT alone during the prodromal period. This finding, however, remains to be replicated. Several carefully performed research studies have documented its efficacy. This treatment is particularly frequently used in the United Kingdom and is now becoming more common by some psychologists in the United States as well.

CBT has two components: behavioral and cognitive. Behavior therapy is supposed to weaken the connections between troublesome situations and an individual's reactions to them. The reactions are such emotions as fear, depression, or rage and other self-defeating or self-damaging behavior. The cognitive aspect of the therapy focuses on changing thought patterns in order to change the emotional state and thus behavior. CBT has been used successfully in conditions such as depression, panic or anxiety disorders, and phobias.

The basis for CBT in schizophrenia is that the disorder consists of a circumscribed set of irrational beliefs, and thus easily learned techniques can alleviate the impact of those beliefs on one's daily life. The CBT therapists work to make patients aware that their thinking patterns are distorted and then train them to change these patterns by a process called "cognitive restructuring." This process is different from psychodynamic psychotherapy, which instead tries to make patients understand why they behave the way they do and assumes that with understanding comes change. CBT does not involve understanding why one behaves a certain way but uses behavior modification techniques to produce change in behavior.

Some techniques used in CBT include behavioral homework assignments that encourage patients to try new responses to difficult situations. Another is called "cognitive rehearsal," where a patient imagines a difficult situation and the therapist guides him or her through dealing with it. Patients may also keep a journal of their thoughts, feelings, and actions, although this may be difficult for patients with schizophrenia. The therapist also will use conditioning (positive reinforcement) and systematic desensitization from fears. Treatment is relatively short in comparison to some other forms of psychotherapy, usually lasting no longer than 16 weeks. Although many insurance plans provide reimbursement for cognitive behavioral therapy services, they may not yet reimburse for this treatment in schizophrenia.

Several organizations specialize in CBT in the United States, including:

- Albert Ellis Institute (formerly the Institute for Rational-Emotive Therapy)
  Address: 45 East 65th Street, New York, NY 10021
  Phone: 1-800-323-4738
  Web site: www.rebt.org
- Beck Institute
  Address: GSB Building, City Line and Belmont Avenues, Suite 700, Bala Cynwyd, PA 19004-1610
  Phone: 1-610-664-3020
  Web site: www.beckinstitute.org
- National Association of Cognitive-Behavioral Therapists
  Address: P.O. Box 2195, Weirton, WV 26062
  Phone: 1-800-853-1135
  Web site: www.nacbt.org

In the United Kingdom, Dr. Douglas Turkington at the University of Newcastle upon Tyne and Dr. Til Wykes at the Institute of Psychiatry in London, as well as others, have written books on this topic (e.g., Kingdon & Turkington, 1995, Reeder and Wykes, 2005). More and more therapists are learning these techniques today, and thus almost every metropolitan area in the United States will have someone available who is practicing CBT.

Beyond CBT, cognitive remediation, in general, can also be helpful for patients who have had comorbid traumatic brain injuries or for post-traumatic stress disorder. Schizophrenia itself is now known to be associated with cognitive deficits. Thus any kind of cognitive training program can be of great benefit for better functioning and quality of life.

35. What can TMS do?

Transcranial magnetic stimulation (TMS) is a new treatment that has gained much popularity recently and has shown proven efficacy for suppressing persistent active auditory hallucinations. TMS utilizes an electromagnet placed on the scalp that generates magnetic field pulses roughly the strength of an MRI (magnetic resonance imaging) scan. The magnetic pulses stimulate a small area on the surface of the brain about the size of a quarter. Low-frequency (once per second) TMS has been shown to induce small, sustained reductions in activity in the part of the brain that has been stimulated. If the part of the temporal lobes thought to be active in auditory hallucinations is stimulated, studies have shown that active hallucinations cease, at least temporarily.

TMS is a novel treatment that is certainly worth trying for resistant hallucinations, although currently not many physicians offer it as a treatment because they have not yet invested in the required equipment. More studies will also be needed to determine whether enough treatments over a period of time can permanently suppress the hallucinations or continued application will be needed. Finally, the side effects of this treatment, because it is so new, are not yet clear.

36. Can a specific diet help?

Unfortunately, throughout the years, there have been proponents of the idea that something in the diet (e.g., too much sugar, too much gluten, aspartame, and pesticides sprayed on field-grown food, or not enough **fish oils**) could cause schizophrenia. Popular organizations stressed that dietary changes would rid the body of toxins, and they encouraged patients with schizophrenia, unfortunately, to discontinue neuroleptic medications. Families would often, out of desperation, turn to these organizations, particularly when their relative was in a particularly severe state and control by medication was difficult. These organizations have been dangerous because they propose plans that have not been substantiated by rigorous research studies or treatment trials. You can today find many Web sites that encourage these alternative treatments.

Fish oil

Omega-3 fatty acids. These substances are important for the building of the lining of nerves. For good functioning of the nervous system, it is important that these fatty acids are in abundance.

37. What about vitamins and fish oil?

Celebrities, who serve as role models, unfortunately are also prone to trying these unconventional treatments and publicizing them. For example, Margot Kidder, the movie star who acted in the *Superman* series, had a severe highly publicized psychotic episode several years ago that led her to become homeless for a while. She claims that medications were not the answer for her. Recently, she appeared on a well-known television talk show recounting how vitamin and mineral therapies have made her symptom free and that Dr. Hoffer, who introduced her to this, saved her life. Dr. Abram Hoffer is well known for his vitamin cocktails that have never been substantiated with scientific treatment trials. Nevertheless, he maintained a faithful following for many years in Saskatchewan, Canada. Large doses of vitamin B_3 (niacin) are the mainstay of his treatment, based on the knowledge that niacin is converted to nicotinamide adenine dinucleotide, an important coenzyme for facilitating various metabolic processes in the body. Niacin also has antihistaminic (antiallergen) properties. Thus, Hoffer's assumption is that "brain allergies" are responsible to some degree for schizophrenic behavior. Part of his regime is a reduced sugar and junk-food diet, which he says requires more niacin to metabolize. He also claims that schizophrenic patients make a substance in their brain that serves as an endogenous hallucinogen and that niacin serves to reduce this toxin in the body. To summarize, no scientific studies can substantiate any of Dr. Hoffer's claims. In general, substituting this treatment regime for neuroleptic medication does more harm than good for people with schizophrenia.

Another recognized pioneer in this field was David Horrobin, who died a few years ago. His area of research had been the clinical use of gamma-linolenic acid (GLA), an omega-3 derivative of an essential oil. It is present in the evening primrose, borage, and black currant seeds. He was one of the first to claim benefits from GLA in treating disease conditions of the nervous system. During his lifetime, he founded Scotia Pharmaceuticals and later Laxdale, Ltd., in Scotland and the journals *Medical Hypotheses* and *Prostaglandins, Leukotrienes, and Essential Fatty Acids*. He was an energetic promoter of evening primrose oil in the treatment of schizophrenia and represented his company in campaigning vigorously for senior renowned scientists to conduct trials of its use. To date, some small studies suggest that it might be weakly beneficial as an adjunct to conventional medication in persons who do not completely respond to their normal treatment regime. Many studies fail to find such an effect. His own controversial trials were under way when he developed a malignant lymphoma, from which he died in 2003. He was an extremely engaging and convincing personality who has had little following to explore his hypotheses further since his untimely death.

38. Can psychotherapy help?

Many types of **psychotherapy** are available, such as supportive, insight oriented, group, and family therapies. The major reason for individuals to consider psychotherapy is that they are unable to help themselves to make progress functioning satisfactorily with family and friends and in an occupation and they would like to improve their quality of life. People with schizophrenia benefit most from help with practical issues. Group therapy can be not only a helpful mechanism to improve one's condition but a social measure as well. The most useful type of therapy to these patients supplements long-term neuroleptic medication and guides the patient in strengthening the complexity of his or her daily activities. Learning how to reach attainable goals through positive reinforcement and encouragement is far more useful than insight-oriented psychodynamic therapy, which is more important for nonpsychotic individuals. Often this therapeutic setting can be provided best by psychiatric social workers.

Psychotherapy
A trained professional talking to a patient in ways that either help provide insight into his/her actions or support and encouragement to deal with life's problems.

39. Can family therapy help?

Family therapy grew out of the many psychodynamic treatments that reached their peak in the 1970s. Two main principles were involved: The first is that there were communication disturbances within the family that led to confusion in the affected individual and which resulted in the symptoms of schizophrenia, and the second is that the patient is not the individual brought for treatment but rather the family unit as a whole. In general, the family therapy movement has caused a lot of damage to the well-being of families and to the relationship between the caregivers and consumers. Parents were told (or at least it was implied) that they were somehow at fault, and they did

Family therapy
A type of treatment that focuses on alleviating problems the entire family entity has interacting with each other. It can also provide support to families having a member with schizophrenia so that members are better able to deal with his/her illness.

not want to be blamed. They needed help to deal with all the management issues that occur when a family member has a serious mental illness. Thus, this type of therapy strained the relationship between families and the medical community, and it has taken many years to regain the trust that is needed for families to support the pharmacotherapy given by psychiatrists that is essential to treat those individuals with schizophrenia.

40. Is electroconvulsive therapy used for schizophrenia?

Electroconvulsive therapy (ECT)

A series of electrical shocks to regions of the brain. Treatment is given in sessions that are separated by several days. It is not dangerous or painful and is accompanied by an anesthesia when administered. Some memory loss subsequent to the treatment can be a side effect. It is mainly used for depression, but can produce temporary improvement in schizophrenia, particularly in people who have persistent painful thoughts and hallucinations.

Electroconvulsive therapy (ECT) has received bad press over the years for its use as a treatment for both schizophrenia and depression. Some hospitals do not allow it, and doctors' privileges to use it are separate from their regular medical licenses and hospital privileges. Certainly, if this is a recommended treatment, the qualifications for the person performing the ECT should be researched and the anesthesiologist as well. This procedure, with anticonvulsant medication given at the same time, is actually quite safe. Controversy exists, however, as to its efficacy for schizophrenia. Most studies do not show clear long-term results and certainly do not indicate that the patient will not have a recurrence even if the acute episode subsides. Maintenance antipsychotic medication will then need to be given. However, one of the reasons to give ECT rather than antipsychotic medication as the first treatment of choice is to avoid the side effects of medication. This is less of an issue now with the advent of the newer medications that have relatively minimal side effects. One side effect of ECT is memory loss, and whether this loss is permanent is unclear. ECT is more commonly given as the last resort in patients with schizophrenia when they have particularly comorbid depressive, manic, or violent symptoms that do not respond to usual medications.

Max Fink (1999), a well-known authority on ECT, has written a helpful book about its uses. In it he describes the beneficial effect of ECT for what he calls "the thought disorders"—the delusional and hallucinatory and language disorganization symptoms that occur predominantly in schizophrenia—but also in other illnesses as well. The number of ECT treatments (as many as 15 to 25), however, that is needed to alleviate these symptoms is larger than that for depression, and it may take longer for the ECT to reach its effect. In addition, if a course of ECT is not repeated, then relapse often occurs. A minimum of 6 months of treatment is recommended (Fink, 1999). Thus, the failure of ECT for schizophrenia that psychiatrists and families perceive could actually be due to a lack of continued treatment.

A combination of ECT and antipsychotic medication may be more efficacious than either alone. Dr. Fink describes the mechanism as one in which the ECT can increase the ability for the medication to enter the neuronal cell membranes and thus exert its physiologic effect. The patient then might also require a smaller dose of the medication and be less likely to experience its side effects. Nevertheless, few psychiatrists use ECT today for schizophrenia, and they are generally not taught to do so in their medical school or residency training.

41. What are the pros and cons of participating in research studies?

Many of the major academic institutions have psychiatrists who conduct research on schizophrenia. Currently, relatively little is known about this disease compared with most other medical disorders; thus, research of multiple kinds needs to continue, with adequate funding from public sources. Although many theories about schizophrenia exist, at present there is no biologic test for it, there are no symptoms that are specific to schizophrenia, and there is no preventive measure one can take to avoid getting this illness. We only know that it has an inherited component of some sort and that it appears usually in early adulthood or late adolescence, that it has some sex differences, and that medications can suppress the symptoms, such as having delusionary perceptions and auditory hallucinations, as long as these medications are taken continuously as prescribed.

Research is desperately needed to find drugs that target the cause of illness and to find treatments that prevent the chronic course before it begins. Research is also needed to find measures to improve the quality of life in those people who develop a chronic illness and are only marginally able to exist outside of an institution. Participating in research studies generally does not help the individual directly but can, in the future, benefit others who develop the illness. However, being in a research study often means that better care is available to the participant and to his or her family because the researchers are generally well recognized as experts in their field and will know where and how to obtain the best treatment, although this is not always the case. Access to care is then facilitated, and earlier detection may result for other family members that can lead to a better outcome.

Participating in research studies generally does not help the individual directly but can, in the future, benefit others who develop the illness.

The NIMH often lists various research studies on its Web site (www.nimh.nih.gov). Researchers advertise through clinics, hospitals, and support groups such as NAMI; if you would like to be part of some of these studies, which are generally not risky, this should be possible. In addition, the rights of individuals who participate in research are protected by an oversight human subjects institutional review board (IRB). Review boards approve written research protocols and stress that the subjects must be competent to provide written informed consent—that is, they must understand the risks and benefits of the research procedures before participating and understand that it is voluntary and they may withdraw without having their clinical treatment with the most established treatments affected. Many years ago, research had the potential to be abusive because there were no laws to govern how it could be done. These practices have changed considerably over the past couple of decades, and how research can be performed in an ethical manner is now a very sensitive issue internationally.

PART THREE

The Consideration of Nongenetic Risk Factors

Do birth complications cause schizophrenia?

Is schizophrenia more common in some cultural or racial groups than others?

Can bad family relationships cause schizophrenia?

More . . .

"The mystique of science proclaims that numbers are the ultimate test of objectivity. Surely we can weigh a brain or score an intelligence test without recording our social preferences. If ranks are displayed in hard numbers obtained by rigorous and standardized procedures, then they must reflect reality, even if they confirm what we want to believe from the start. . . . If quantitative data are as subject to cultural constraint as any other aspect of science, then they have no special claim upon final truth."

—Stephen Jay Gould, *The Mismeasure of Man*, 1981

42. Do birth complications cause schizophrenia?

Prenatal

The period between conception and birth.

Hippocampus

A relatively small brain structure that lies deep within the temporal lobe and is thought to be crucial for memory. It has been given this name because of its unusual curved shape.

Numerous studies on the association of obstetric complications (both **prenatal** and perinatal) with schizophrenia have been reported over the years. No single specific complication has been implicated, however, in causing schizophrenia. Birth complications considered in the studies have included bleeding during pregnancy, influenza during the second trimester, premature birth, and excessively long labor. Some investigators have hypothesized that many birth complications lead to transient hypoxia to the developing brain, and when occurring at a particular stage in development, the later fully developed brain will be more vulnerable to schizophrenia. Particularly, it is thought that the cells of the **hippocampus** are most vulnerable to perinatal complications, such that its growth may be suppressed during a crucial period. These are just theories without proof, and, in fact, some good studies now show no association of later schizophrenia with having been born with birth complications. At least one study of siblings with and without schizophrenia shows that they have no difference in frequency of having had birth complications. Thus, how can one draw conclusions about these data? First, the studies examining birth complications use various methods for selecting control individuals for comparison and for obtaining a history of birth complications. Controls need to be matched for social class and sex. When this is done by comparison to well siblings for an example, the association with birth complications is less clear. Similarly, taking an obstetric history from mothers is fraught with bias, as it has been shown that mothers tend to remember more birth complications occurring in their chronically ill offspring than in those who are well.

Stronger studies result from prospective analyses of large birth cohorts where data have been archived systematically from birth. Several of these studies in the United Kingdom and the United States have been published with equivocal results overall. Given that the vast majority of adults who were born after prenatal complications *do not* develop schizophrenia, it is suspected that these are not significant risk factors for schizophrenia. Mothers who suffer such complications should not have to worry that in the future their child will be any more likely to develop schizophrenia than the child's peers. Pediatricians should not be warning of such.

Given that the vast majority of adults who were born after prenatal complications do not *develop schizophrenia, it is suspected that these are not significant risk factors for schizophrenia.*

43. Is schizophrenia more common in some cultural or racial groups than others?

The answer to this question is most likely no. Stephen Jay Gould in his book *The Mismeasure of Man* showed that seemingly objective quantitative data can be erroneously associated with the wrong characteristics due to societal bias, such as in the association of head size and intelligence (see the quote at the beginning of Part 3). Some studies have associated schizophrenia with lower socioeconomic status, and in some countries, this diagnosis appears more frequently in one racial or cultural group rather than another. The reasons for these inconsistencies are many and include the tendency of physicians to diagnose schizophrenia rather than other forms of psychosis in persons who do not communicate well because their culture or language is different from the physician's or because it is not understood well. For example, in some religious sects in the United States and other countries, services become highly emotional with chanting that can give some people the appearance of being acutely psychotic, as people are "communicating with God." In some cultures, paranoia may be justified given the political history that some individuals have experienced. The examples can go on.

Nevertheless, the World Health Organization has conducted multicenter incidence studies to show that schizophrenia is present throughout the world at relatively similar incidence rates across many different cultures. Other reports indicate its presence in Papua New Guinea (despite previous reports to the contrary), the Australian aboriginals, and the isolated ancient San population of South Africa. In fact, schizophrenia is possibly present in every population of the world because its origins are as old as the origins of modern Homo sapiens themselves. One great thinker on schizophrenia (Crow, 1997) describes schizophrenia as "the price Homo sapiens pays for language," meaning that schizophrenia is at the extreme of the uniquely human genetic variation that distinguishes modern human beings from all other primates and that gave us the ability to communicate by complex language.

Nevertheless, many disparities do exist in the diagnosis and treatment of schizophrenia across ethnic and racial groups. These issues are sensitive, but their underlying bases need to be better understood. Rather than being fuel for stigmatizing groups, the differences, whether they be socially or biologically induced, need to be recognized so that each group may be better served with individualized treatments as needed.

44. Can bad family relationships cause schizophrenia?

An emphatic answer to this question is *no*, and this myth must be dispelled. Several years ago it was popular among psychiatrists and psychologists to presume that the cause of schizophrenia had to do with poor mothering, or the "schizophrenogenic mother," as the term became coined. These mothers were supposedly giving mixed messages to their child, causing pathologic ambivalence and confusion. This notion, however, was not based on any carefully controlled research studies, but rather on subjective observations of some senior well-respected psychodynamically oriented psychiatrists of the time. Another set of researchers introduced the term *expressed emotion* to the field and produced data to suggest that the greater the expressed emotion in a family, the more likely a psychosis would develop in an individual. These data, however, were refuted by others who argued that higher expressed emotion in any family with a schizophrenic member may have more to do with the frustration the family feels having to deal with a chronically ill individual who can cause frequent serious crises by virtue of the disorder itself. At best, one can say that a kind, reassuring, protective, and supportive intact family will aid someone afflicted with schizophrenia to have a better outcome to his or her illness than a disruptive and unsupportive family environment.

In the 1960s the concept that schizophrenia was due to miscommunication among members of a nuclear family was a very popular concept. The mother, who had a more intense interaction with the child from infancy on, was considered to be the one who had the most influence and most chance to transmit miscommunications that were termed "schizophrenogenic." A famous analyst, Frieda-Fromm Reichmann, was known to espouse the theory of regressing patients back to infancy and then bringing them back to their current age with a particular kind of analysis that claimed to recreate the mothering that was never received. Unfortunately, this concept has caused much harm to families and their relationships with psychiatrists trying to treat the patient. Currently, no scientific basis suggests that a mother's communication style is harmful to a young child and can cause later schizophrenia.

45. Can immigration from another country increase risk for schizophrenia?

Some very interesting studies in the United Kingdom and the Netherlands have shown that Afro-Caribbeans and other migrant groups to foreign countries have an increase of schizophrenia in themselves and their offspring after having arrived in a foreign culture. Currently, the cause of this phenomenon is unclear—that is, whether it is genetic or environmental or an artifact of the data collection. The difficulties of adjusting to life in a foreign country economically and socially can certainly provide fertile ground for the development of all kinds of emotional problems in later life. Despite these reports, the vast majority of immigrants to new lands do not develop schizophrenia. One could comment that countries such as the United States and Australia, made up by a majority of different waves of immigrant groups over time, have not reported increases in schizophrenia as a result.

46. Is it better to live in a rural area?

Some epidemiologic surveys have found that schizophrenia appears more prevalent in urban than rural areas within the same country. Similarly, the prevalence of schizophrenia may be less, although the incidence is the same, in underdeveloped rather than developed industrialized countries. This finding may be comparable to the urban versus rural distinction. Reasons for this disparity could be many and may have to do with the outcome of acute psychotic episodes. In general, rural and nonindustrialized environments tend to have extended families living together or close by, and thus emotional support for psychotic individuals is greater. These individuals also tend to be tolerated more in these environments and have more space to be alone so that they do not need to interact by force with others. It would be easier to stay out of a hospital or treatment facility existing in such environments. Recovery might be seen as a nonviolent, quiet behavior, and the inner world of someone with schizophrenia would not only be more tolerable but less noticeable. This does not mean, however, that it is better to live in a rural area if you have schizophrenia! Urban environments tend to provide patients with better medical care, more available psychiatrists and related healthcare personnel, and better access to the newest treatments.

47. Is schizophrenia infectious?

Once a curious Russian physician, who reported the results from an epidemiological survey of dwellings in Moscow, claimed that clusters of schizophrenia occurred in specific neighborhoods (Kasanetz, 1979). Torrey (1980), in his book *Schizophrenia and Civilization*, claims that pockets of schizophrenia exist in counties of Ireland, suggesting that schizophrenia could be infectious or spread from one individual to another. Crow and Done (1986), however, in a landmark analysis of a large number of pairs of siblings with schizophrenia, showed that despite two siblings living together, the time of onset of their illness was not correlated, although their age of onset was. If an illness is contagious, one expects that two people living together would get it relatively close in time. If they seem to get the illness at the same age, the onset is predetermined by other factors such as developmental and/or genetic ones. Thus, the infectious theory "holds no water" and has largely been abandoned.

48. Do viruses cause schizophrenia?

An infectious agent may cause an illness, however, without being directly infectious. Dating back to Menninger in the early 1900s, there was a suspicion that viruses could cause schizophrenia. As Karl Menninger noted (1926), the great influenza epidemic of 1918 saw an increase of schizophrenia admissions to hospitals. Through the years since, particularly revived by Torrey and Peterson (1976), the viral hypothesis of schizophrenia has carried weight among some researchers even today. Many viral infections have been implicated besides influenza, such as cytomegalovirus, herpes I and II, Epstein-Barr virus, toxoplasmosis, and some uniquely human retroviruses. The positive findings from these studies, however, have not been consistently replicated, and no active viral particles have ever been definitively isolated from the brains of people with schizophrenia after death. One of the more prevalent theories about these viruses is that a mother acquires the infection during the second trimester of pregnancy, a crucial time for brain higher cortical center development, making offspring more vulnerable to develop schizophrenia in later life. This is just a theory for which there is not yet convincing substantiating evidence.

PART FOUR

The Genetic Risk

Is schizophrenia inherited, and if so, how?

If I have a brother with schizophrenia and my partner does too, what are the chances of our children getting schizophrenia?

How has biologic genetic research on schizophrenia been conducted in the past?

More . . .

"Mendel had painstakingly backcrossed pollen and egg cells from the common pea plant to reach a better understanding of inheritance. Mendel had recorded . . . his findings in a two-part lecture in 1865 . . . and then was all but ignored for the rest of his life . . . but rediscovered by Bateson in May 1900. Nearly a century after the debate over Mendelism that set the stage for contemporary genetics, almost every part of our modern understanding of how the world works—the relationship between parent and offspring . . . and the commonalities among all living things—can in a large measure be traced back to that startling spring of 1900, when anything was possible."

—Robin Marantz Henig, *The Monk in the Garden,* 2000

49. What are the lessons from history?

The ideas of genes, genetics, and specific patterns of inheritance grew out of the discoveries of the late 1800s and early 1900s, and thus the field of genetics was born, gradually evolving into what we know of its science today. With it, however, also grew the notion of eugenics (i.e., if genetic defects caused undesirable traits, one could eliminate these traits in society). Sterilization became an acceptable procedure for people who were considered "misfits" in society and included those with mental retardation and also psychiatric disturbances in state institutions even in the USA. Although little is publicized about these times, the Cold Spring Harbor Laboratories (Long Island, New York), today a center of excellence in molecular genetics, was in its earlier years a hotbed in the United States for the eugenics movement.

The Holocaust of the mid-twentieth century looms high on the list of human atrocities in recent times. It was characterized by a program for the extermination of people for the sole reason that their heritage included Jewish ancestry. However, less is publicized about the considerable participation of German psychiatrists at that time in the extermination of psychotic patients in psychiatric hospitals. In Germany alone, at least five main such hospitals were equipped with gas chambers and connected incinerators during the years 1938 to 1940. Preservation of the building for such procedures can be seen today in the Hadamar Psychiatric Hospital, a short distance from Frankfurt, where a museum depicts the scene of busloads of patients being delivered each day down to the "showers" by one door and then out the opposite door as corpses to the autopsy table for the academic neuropathologist/psychiatrist to examine the postmortem brain before incineration. Eventually, but not before 10,000 patients were exterminated in this way at Hadamar, the Bishop of Muenster spoke out about this suspected atrocity, and Hitler was forced to abandon this effort in the psychiatric hospitals. Nevertheless, the doctors and nurses continued various methods of euthanasia by injection and starvation until the end of World War II and the fall of the Nazi party. This is a striking example of the extreme misuse of genetic information. One may simply read this and say that it cannot happen again and that perhaps the lesson from history has been learned. But has it?

We are part of a different scientific age now. The explosion of new technology in the field of genetics has enabled us to identify variations in almost all genes in the human genome. What will be done with this information now that we have it needs continual discussion and legislation. The science-fiction movie *Gattaca* produced in 1997 is an example of what could go wrong, or is wrong. Two classes of human beings were depicted in this movie: those whose genes were "enhanced" in utero (i.e., deleterious variants were replaced with "better" ones) and those who were born of natural unions between men and women. The latter were discriminated against, could not get professional jobs, and were forbidden to marry

What will be done with this information now that we have it needs continual discussion and legislation.

those who were enhanced. Everyone carried his or her own **deoxyribonucleic acid (DNA)** card, which was proof of his or her identity. Could this happen in reality?

Deoxyribonucleic acid (DNA)

Inherited material made of different nucleic acids put together in the form of a triple helix. It consists of a long polymer with a deoxyribose and phosphate backbone and four different bases: adenine, guanine, cytosine, and thymine. Genes are made up of DNA and the variation in genes between individuals depends on the sequence of these nucleic acids in an individual's genes. Chromosomes are made up of sequences of DNA with genes intermittently spaced along the chromosome and separated by segments of DNA that do not represent an inherited function (or genes). DNA makes up the chromosomes of all animals and plants and many viruses.

Scientifically, no barriers exist. Already in vitro fertilization allows parents to choose the eye and hair color for a baby and unlimited other characteristics of their choice. Commercial companies, such as *23 and Me,* exist to give consumers a look at what they have inherited in their own genome. What we do with new genetic information must be open for serious discussion.

50. Is schizophrenia inherited, and if so, how?

On April 14, 1930, four identical quadruplets weighing from 3 to 4.5 pounds were born by natural birth after a short labor and were placed in incubators. Although their childhood achievements varied, they grew up close and with much societal attention until within 6 months of each other in their early adulthood, they all had acute psychotic episodes eventually diagnosed as schizophrenia. Their notoriety as four identical individuals who all had schizophrenia led to their being brought to the NIMH Laboratory of Psychology in the 1950s to be studied by a well-known group of investigators interested in searching for the causes of schizophrenia and particularly in pursuing the gene environment or nature-versus-nurture controversy. Every test in use at that time, from the Rorschach to conventional **electroencephalograms (EEGs)**, was given to the quadruplets. The investigators, David Rosenthal and Seymour Kety, first director of NIMH, went on from there to design adoption studies to be conducted in Denmark and produced pioneering data that turned the thinking of the time around from environmental to genetic/biologic causes.

Electroencephalogram (EEG)

A type of test whereby electrodes are placed on several areas of the head and recordings are made of the brain's electrical activity.

There were also studies of twins at NIMH, such as those by David Shakow, which led to many theories about environment and development of people who get schizophrenia. David Rosenthal, however, was the one that particularly developed a relationship with the family of the quadruplets, giving them the name "Genain," meaning "bad blood," and pseudonyms Nora, Iris, Myrna, and Hester (representing NIMH) so that he could publish his findings but maintain the family's privacy.

Again, in 1979, after publication of the Kety–Rosenthal adoption studies and international recognition of the implications of these results, the Genains, then almost 50 years old, were brought back to NIMH to the laboratory of neuropsychopharmacology, to be examined for abnormalities in all of the biologic markers that were claimed to be important for schizophrenia at the time. I was privileged to be a young postdoctoral fellow in charge of managing the procedures and caring for these women during their 2-month stay on the inpatient research ward. At that time David Rosenthal accompanied them to NIMH but quickly remained in the background, dealing with his own newly diagnosed Alzheimer's disease. During the period of getting to know these women, their fears, and variety of similar delusions and hallucinations, I also came to know the kind, silent face of Dr. Rosenthal, whose personal copy of his book, *The Genain Quadruplets*, was later taken off his office shelf and presented to me for my service to the Genains in his absence. Whether we learned anything useful from working intensely with the Genains during that period was questionable, but the experience left a deep impression in my memory—no family can have such bad luck as to have four of four children with schizophrenia unless the illness is genetic. My later mentor in psychiatric genetics, Elliot S. Gershon, remarked during that time that I had gotten myself an "N of one," meaning essentially only one case study, nothing more, because these women all shared identical DNA sequences, and that nothing of any scientific rigor could come out of such a genetic comparison study; rather, I needed to study many more such families. Of course, he was ahead of the times and was correct, already a pioneer himself in more fruitful genetic research.

The thought that schizophrenia is inherited dates back to early twentieth-century descriptions of the condition (see *Dementia Praecox* by Emil Kraepelin). Kraepelin (1907) estimated that "defective heredity," as he called it, was prominent and present in over 70% of cases. From his early writings on, large family studies were conducted throughout Europe, particularly to estimate the amount of illness in close family members of individuals with schizophrenia. In general, they were consistent with the notion that there was an excess risk for schizophrenia to close relatives (siblings, offspring) of approximately 10% but that the risks fell dramatically in more distant relatives, such as aunts, uncles, and cousins (**Table 1**). The highest risks, however, were shown to be present in **monozygotic twin** pairs based on a series of independent twin studies. The biggest dilemma in psychiatric genetics today, however, is the attempt to explain why, although the risk to monozygotic twins is highest of any recorded risk factor for schizophrenia, it falls considerably short of 100% (i.e., only 50% on average), which is the percentage you would expect if two individuals share an identical genetic makeup. Although most people seem to think that this low concordance rate among identical twins is evidence for environmental interactions, modification of genes by internally controlled molecular mechanisms has

Monozygotic twins

Twins born at the same time who originate from the splitting of the same egg after it has been fertilized. The DNA is identical in both twins; and thus the twins are sometimes referred to as identical.

Table 1 Familial Risks for Schizophrenia in Relatives of People with Schizophrenia (Modified from Gottesman II [1991].)

Relationship	% Chance of Developing Schizophrenia	% Chance of Developing an Illness with a Dominant Inheritance
Identical twins	48	100
Nonidentical twins	17	50
Siblings	9	50
Children	13	50
Parents	6	50
Grandchildren	5	25
Nieces and nephews	4	25
Aunts and uncles	2	25
First cousins	2	12.5
Unrelated individuals	1	N/A*

*Dependent on the prevalence of the risk gene in the population.

not been excluded and could alter their expression such that one person of an identical twin-pair could develop a trait or illness, and the other not.

The turning point in schizophrenia research and probably the most important data collection and results of the twentieth century in this field came from the carefully planned and executed adoption studies of Seymour Kety and David Rosenthal using Danish case registries to identify parents with schizophrenia and their offspring (Rosenthal et al., 1968) and adopted-at-birth children who developed schizophrenia, and their biologic and adoptive relatives (Kety et al., 1968). As a group, regardless of the study design, these investigators showed that an excess of schizophrenia was present in the biologic relatives of individuals with schizophrenia, but not the adoptive relatives. These data were fuel for the nature-versus-nurture debates of the time and initiated great changes in the focus of research on schizophrenia from the 1970s to the present. Initially, when these results were reported, the leadership of academic psychiatry departments throughout the United States was predominantly made up of psychoanalysts, as was also true of the most prestigious of training institutes. Soon these individuals, however, were replaced by biologically oriented chairpersons who led a new era of research—and the field of biologic psychiatry was born.

51. If my aunt, uncle, or cousin has schizophrenia, what are the chances of my children getting it?

Your children would share the same amount of genetic material with your parent's siblings as you do with your own first cousin, and the risk for schizophrenia in both cases would be very small and almost the same as in the general population.

We do not know what the real risks are until the actual genes that lead to a predisposition for schizophrenia are identified and their mechanisms for producing disease determined.

52. If I have a brother with schizophrenia and my partner does too, what are the chances of our children getting schizophrenia?

These risks are also small and about 2%. It may be twice that if the illness is present in both sides of the family; the chances of a child becoming affected would be greater, although there are no clear statistics to say how much greater. In addition, these are only general risk statistics, and thus what happens in each individual family will vary. We do not know what the real risks are until the actual genes that lead to a predisposition for schizophrenia are identified and their mechanisms for producing disease determined. The risks shown in

Table 1 are based only on prevalence rates from the old large family studies that exist. Moreover, one has to consider that since the 1980s there have been newer, carefully controlled family studies using the American Psychiatric Association *DSM* diagnostic categories. In these studies, the risk to any close family relative (for example, a sibling or child of an affected person) is still in excess but is considerably lower than in previous reports (on average about 7%–8%).

53. If I have an identical twin with schizophrenia, but I am well, what are my children's chances of having schizophrenia?

According to some twin studies, it appears that the risk for schizophrenia to offspring of well versus ill identical twins is the same and would be similar to the risk to children in general (i.e., 13%; see Table 1). These studies, however, have been flawed in design and limited in their numbers. People with schizophrenia, particularly men, have fewer offspring than those who do not have schizophrenia; thus, the number of offspring of ill versus well identical twins will not likely be the same. Because of the difficulties in obtaining and studying identical twins where one has schizophrenia, the numbers for comparisons in these studies are small. This issue is thus still controversial but is an important one. If these rates were equal, then one assumes that something in the genetic sequence (identical DNA sequence) must be what is crucial for schizophrenia susceptibility. If these rates really are unequal, *although* still in excess in the offspring of the well twin, then some modification of the defective gene's expression, either endogenously or by the environment, is likely to be taking place as well. We hope that molecular genetic studies of twins will yield some answers to this question in the near future.

54. How has biologic genetic research on schizophrenia been conducted in the past?

Before the late 1980s, the biologic research that was pursued on the genetics of schizophrenia was largely conducted by examining factors in blood, urine, and cerebral spinal fluid that were different in chronic patients with schizophrenia compared with controls. Then these factors that were inherited were examined by comparing the similarity in these factors between pairs of identical versus nonidentical twins, the logic being that the environment was the same for these twins, but the genes in nonidentical twins were different. These numerous studies produced nothing consistent, and in fact many of those early positive findings were eventually found to be due to either the medications the patients were taking, their dietary differences, or the effects of institutionalization. They were not found to be inherited when normal sets of twins were compared if those studies were performed. When the field of molecular genetics began to explode in the early 1980s by producing multiple highly variable markers spread throughout the genome for specific genes, it became clear that these markers could be used to map the chromosomal location of different diseases and then, by identifying genes in the specific mapped location, to find a variation in a gene that leads to that specific disease. These methods were then applied to psychiatric disorders with genetic susceptibility, particularly schizophrenia.

Linkage

A genetic term that signifies a relationship between two or more genes on the same chromosome that are relatively close together so that sometimes the variations in the traits that each represents are inherited together in the same individual. When genes are linked in a genetic sense, they are close together on a chromosome and thus the inherited variations in them are more likely than chance to occur together in the same individual.

Chromosome

A structure present in the nucleus of every cell of the body of any living thing and containing genes.

55. What does linkage to a chromosome mean?

Many research groups worldwide began to evaluate families that by virtue of having more than one sibling with schizophrenia were considered ideal for these chromosomal **linkage** studies. The principles of genetic linkage studies are as follows: Our genes are organized in predetermined locations on pairs of 23 **chromosomes**

(46 total). One of each pair is inherited from each parent. During reproduction, however, an independent assortment of the maternal and paternal genes on chromosome pairs exists so that the farther away genes are on each chromosome, the greater the likelihood that different combinations of genes are inherited on the final chromosomes of the offspring of a mother–father pair. This independent assortment is why no two siblings look alike unless they are identical twins and come from the same egg and sperm during fertilization.

If there are known highly variable markers that could be spaced out across all chromosomes, one could then see which variations in the markers are present in each individual and trace the inheritance of variations in these markers down generations in families (**Figure 1**). In each

CHROMOSOME 1 and its variants in markers:

___A,B,C,D,E,F___	___G,H,I,J, K___**SZ**___	___M,N,O___
Marker 1	Marker 2	Marker 3

Typical family pedigree and the inheritance of Marker 2:

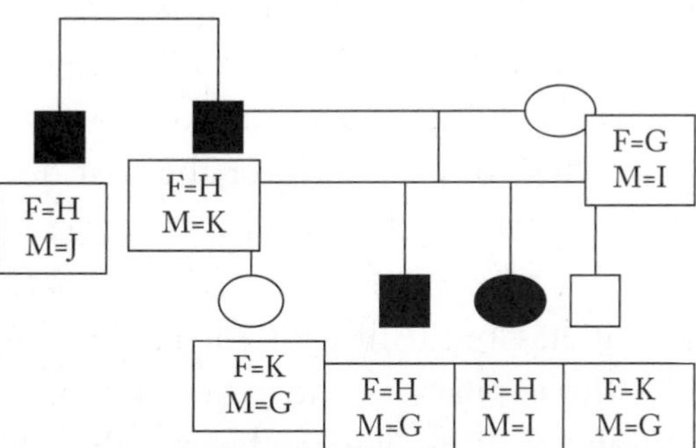

Figure 1 Illustration of linkage of schizophrenia to a chromosome if Marker 2 on chromosome 1 is linked to schizophrenia (SZ). The boxes indicate the variants each person inherited. "F" is from the person's father and "M" is from the person's mother. ■ = has schizophrenia and □ = well. Circles are women and squares are males. Note that the "H" variant of Marker 2 is present in all people who have schizophrenia in this family.

family, different variations in the markers will be present (because the mother has two and the father has two), but it is the position of the markers on chromosomes that is important, not the exact variation in the marker. Think of maps of towns. We have street names that vary and are different. The unique names help us locate houses on the streets. We can find the house because it is located between two named street signs. So it is with a disease gene. It is not the marker itself that will cause an illness, but it is the gene for an illness that is close to a specific marker that is important. If an illness gene is close to that marker, it will tend to be transmitted with the marker down generations, and we then say it is "linked." It is said to be "mapped" near that marker. **Geneticists**, based on this information in families with multiple ill and well members, are able to calculate how likely it is that a gene for illness is linked to a marker, given the pattern of marker inheritance that is observed in families such as the one illustrated in Figure 1. This method has been highly successful in the search to find genes for disorders known to be genetic, such as Huntington's chorea or phenylketonuria.

Geneticists

Scientists who study the inheritance of traits in humans, animals, or plants.

A gene, however, such as one for schizophrenia, may be only one of many that causes the same illness and may have a nontraditional more complex mode of inheritance. Thus it will not be so easy to find by this method. In fact, the irony is that over the past decade there have been reports of many positive linkage findings for schizophrenia spread throughout all 23 chromosomes, and it has been difficult for researchers to tell which of these positives are true findings and which are falsely positive, having been only chance findings. The key to this dilemma will be to find strong gene candidates whose involvement makes sense given their known functions and to corroborate these findings by other sources of evidence.

56. What are the methods developed to find gene functional and structural differences?

The explosion of new technology in molecular genetics in recent years has resulted in the development of **ribonucleic acid (RNA) microarrays** and gene chip microarrays.

Ribonucleic acid (RNA)

A nucleic acid polymer that plays an important role in the process that translates genetic information from DNA into protein products.

Microarray

An orderly arrangement of DNA samples to identify many genes at one time. They can contain thousands of genes on one small plate or "chip." An experiment with a single DNA chip or microarray can provide researchers information on thousands of genes simultaneously. There are also RNA arrays that can provide information about gene expression.

Of all the genetic material in the human genome, only a very small amount of the DNA sequence actually leads to the production of proteins that, in turn, have a function in the body. The DNA that will be expressed is transferred into complementary sequences of messenger RNA (mRNA) that produce proteins critical to directing all bodily functions. This process is called *gene expression*. It is complicated by many control mechanisms that enable the crucial timing of expression of genes and their turning on and off at different times in the life span of individuals.

Gene expression throughout the genome can be examined on microarrays in a direct and comprehensive way, as can gene structural variation among individuals and gene methylation (modification by methyl groups). Gene structure is simply the sequence of nucleic acids along its chain and how it folds. Expression on the other hand has to do with when in the individual the DNA actually is stimulated to produce RNA and then in turn proteins. Microarray technology enables researchers to examine structure and function of thousands of genes at once in the laboratory. The microarrays themselves are small slide or plate-like laboratory structures that support thousands of genes at fixed immobilized locations. The researcher places the genes in these locations in an orderly fashion, and thus, it is called an "array." If the expression of a gene is to be examined, the experiment is called "microarray expression analysis." If a gene is overexpressed in a certain disease state, then more of a sample of a sequence of expressed DNA will be present compared with control DNA. Arrays use fluorescent colors to quantify the amount of expression; if a particular gene expression is involved, it may be seen by expression of a different color. Similarly, the colors are different if structure is examined for different bases or if a segment is or is not methylated.

In schizophrenia research, microarray expression studies have been carried out on postmortem brains of patients who had chronic schizophrenia. Many results have come out of these studies, but it is still too early to tell whether the findings are consistent and relate to the findings from the linkage studies. Some early expression studies implicate genes for neuronal connectivity and growth. These studies, however, have so far not been able to clarify the effects that medication intake and other problems of illness chronicity and aging have on differential gene expression. In addition, examining brains of older people after death may not be useful for finding genes that are expressed only during brain development prenatally and in childhood.

Most recently, microarrays have been used in genome-wide association studies (the GWAS). These studies have used chips coated with as many as a million markers to examine whether a specific common variant is associated with schizophrenia in very large numbers of patients compared with controls (as many as 10,000 or more). The results are so far only initial, and need to be replicated, but at present many of the studies, while reporting significant findings, do not report the same ones and also have surprisingly few significant findings. Of course, this method will reveal important discoveries only if risk genes for schizophrenia are actually common gene variants currently in the population.

57. What are the current candidate genes for schizophrenia?

Before the recent GWAS studies, there were claims from several linkage studies that genes within these regions that are known to be brain expressed could be involved in susceptibility for schizophrenia. The exact nature of their roles has not been elucidated, although some have general relevance particularly to glutamatergic neurochemical brain pathways that appear widespread throughout the brain and have been thought to be relevant to schizophrenia. Others clearly are involved in brain growth during development (**Table 2**).

Table 2 Some Candidates in Linked Chromosomal Regions for Schizophrenia. These genes may play some role in functions that make people more vulnerable for developing schizophrenia. However, at this time, they have not shown to be definitely involved.

	Chromosome Location	Action
Disc I & II	1q	Brain growth
RGS4	1q	Glutamate pathway
Dysbindin	6p	Brain growth
Neuregulin	8p	Brain growth
PPP3CC calcineurin	8p	Calmodulin-dependent protein phosphatase
BDNF	11p	Brain growth
DAO	12q	Glutamate pathway
DAOA	13q	Glutamate pathway
G72	13q	Glutamate pathway
COMT	22q	Dopamine metabolism
PRODH	22q	Oxidative stress
ZDHHC8	22q	Palmitoylation
Synapsin III	22q	Brain development

Aside from linkage and microarray studies, there are the so-called early candidate gene-association studies, where a specific variant in a gene is more frequent in populations of people with schizophrenia than in control populations. Many positive results have also come out of these studies because the standards for what consists of a positive finding have not yet been agreed on by researchers in the field. What is interesting is that these were relatively small studies with positive results. The recent GWAS studies are very large and do not find the same candidate genes. There is much controversy about why this discrepancy exists. Some researchers say that the GWAS studies are flawed in that they do not necessarily cover the regions of the candidate genes that are mentioned in the next paragraph, and would not find them if their effects on risk are present but relatively rare. Some very recent GWAS have revealed a potential candidate near the HLA immune gene-complex on chromosome 6p. This finding needs further examination.

Copy number variation (CNV)

A CNV is a segment of DNA in which a difference in the number of copies of sequences has been found by comparing DNA from two or more people. These may be inherited or caused by de novo mutations. CNVs are common throughout each person's genome. Sometimes if they occur within genes, they may change their function and could be pathologic.

The following are the major genes that have been associated with schizophrenia by one method or another. What should be clear, however, is that no pathological defect has been found in any of these genes—that is, a mutation has not been found in people with schizophrenia and not in controls, with the possible exception of one or two reports in single rare families and the rare **copy number variations (CNVs)** in some families that are described later. For the most part, however, these studies have not shown that within multiple families all those with schizophrenia have the putative variant, whereas those who do not have schizophrenia do not have the variant. The list of putative candidates includes brain-derived neurotrophic factor (BDNF), B-37, ciliary neurotrophic factor (CNTF), CNPase, COMT, DBH, DRD2, DRD3, DRD4, DISC I and DISC II, Dysbindin, 14-3-3-eta gene, G-72, G(olf), HSKCa3, HOPA, 5HT2a receptor, KCNH2, MAO-A and MAO-B, MAG, MAL, mGluR, MOG, neuregulin-1, nicotinic cholinergic receptor-a (CHRNA2), NOGO, NOTCH, PIP5K2A, PPP3CC (Calcineurin), proline oxidase, PRODH, RGS proteins, synapsin-III, synapsin-IIIa, TNF-a, tyrosine hydroxylase, and ZDHHC8. Presently, many, if not all, of these claimed genes could be false-positive research findings. Definitive replication studies are urgently needed.

58. *What do DNA copy number variations (CNVs) have to do with schizophrenia?*

One theory is that the genetic mechanism for schizophrenia could be due to multiple rare mutations throughout the genome in genes relevant to brain growth and development or functioning. These mutations can either be inherited from parent to offspring or arise from a so-called mutational hotspot in the genome and spontaneously occur in the germline for one individual.

One theory is that the genetic mechanism for schizophrenia could be due to multiple rare mutations throughout the genome in genes relevant to brain growth and development or functioning.

This theory has been borne out recently with the discovery that there are numerous segments that are duplicated throughout the genome in every person. **Segmental duplications** are sections of DNA with near-identical sequence in the human genome (**Figure 2**). Between these segments are genes. When maternal and paternal chromosomes come together during meiosis to form an embryo, the segments disrupt the proper pairing of chromosomes and either regions of genes are duplicated along the chromosome of the embryo or they are deleted. These microduplications or deletions have been dubbed "copy number variations," or CNVs, and the gene or genes involved may be malfunctioning or disrupted as a result. A significant increase in CNVs has been reported in the genome of people with schizophrenia in some recent

Segmental duplications

Repeats of segments of DNA sequences along a chromosome.

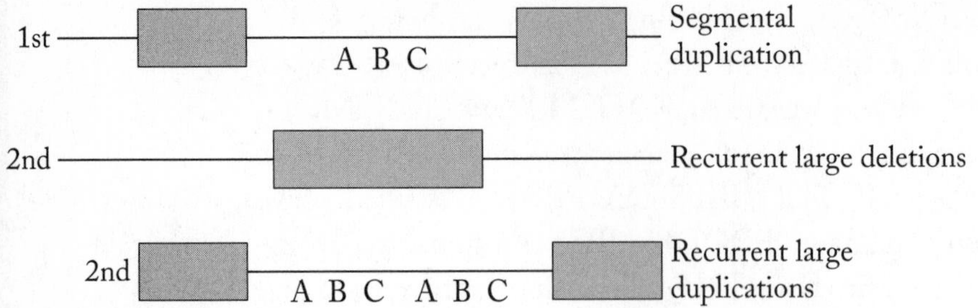

Figure 2 Segmental Duplications and Copy Number Variations. The line represents one chromosome; ABC = 3 different genes or portions of genes along the chromosome. 1st = 1st generation; 2nd = what may occur in offspring as a result of the segmental duplication. Either the region in between with genes A,B, and C is deleted or it is duplicated after recombination of maternal and paternal chromosomes to form the embryo.

large studies, and some specific regions of the genome where they exist have been implicated. However, these studies are still in their infancy. It is not known what the pattern of CNVs is like within families that have members with schizophrenia, and this needs to be studied.

59. How is it assumed that genes cause schizophrenia?

Neuronal transmission is maintained by complex interaction of several neurochemicals with specific receptors on nerve cells. These neurochemicals include dopamine, serotonin, GABA (gamma-aminobutyric acid), norepinephrine, glutamate, and acetylcholine. Because schizophrenia and other serious psychiatric disorders can be controlled by changing the balance of different neurotransmitters, specific receptors have become targets for the development of pharmacotherapies—i.e., new drugs, many of which have mixed profiles for how they affect multiple types of receptors. However, because a drug may suppress the illness by blocking a specific receptor, it does not suggest that the receptor is necessarily responsible for the illness. In fact, while most of the effective treatments for schizophrenia involve blocking dopamine D_2 receptors, the genes for these receptors have not been found to be associated with schizophrenia. Some general trends, however, have been noticed about the way candidate genes particularly converge on the neurochemical pathways for the nervous system nerve transmitter **glutamate**. Others, however, appear to have functions involved in developing neuronal structural networks, such as in aiding the migration of neurons during growth of the brain.

Glutamine/ glutamate

An amino acid that is a building block of proteins. It is also by itself one of the major neurotransmitters in the brain (i.e., transmits information from cell to cell); by stimulating the activity of the cells, it excites them into activity.

One possible scenario is that one or more genes are defective in a certain way and that these genes are turned on and off during different stages of an individual's life span, perhaps even in an abnormal timing mechanism as well. Thus, during prenatal development, some brain structures may develop abnormally in a subtle way; during adolescence, neuronal connections may abnormally form; and during aging, neurons may age in an accelerated or abnormal way. Decreased brain plasticity will result (**Figure 3**). All this is caused

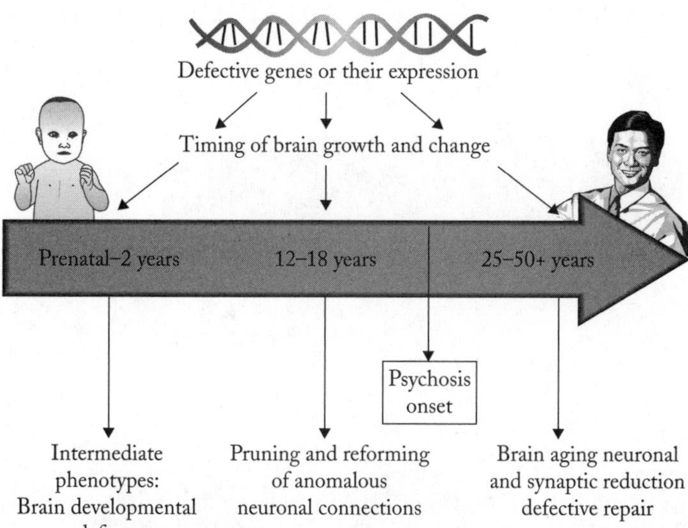

Figure 3 Schizophrenia is a lifetime disorder with different genetically controlled events occurring at each stage by activation and deactivation of the same defective genes. Thus, schizophrenia can be both a neurodevelopmental disorder as well as degenerative with progressive changes deviating from normal after the onset of illness.

by abnormalities in one or more genes and/or their expression at different times during life.

60. What is an intermediate phenotype (sometimes called endophenotype) for schizophrenia?

It is now thought that genes that cause schizophrenia likely act by affecting an "intermediate step"—that is, directly cause a change in the brain that will then, in combination with other things, lead to a vulnerability for developing schizophrenia. In this theory, the genetic defects themselves are not directly responsible for the illness as a whole (**Figure 4**). The rules for what is an

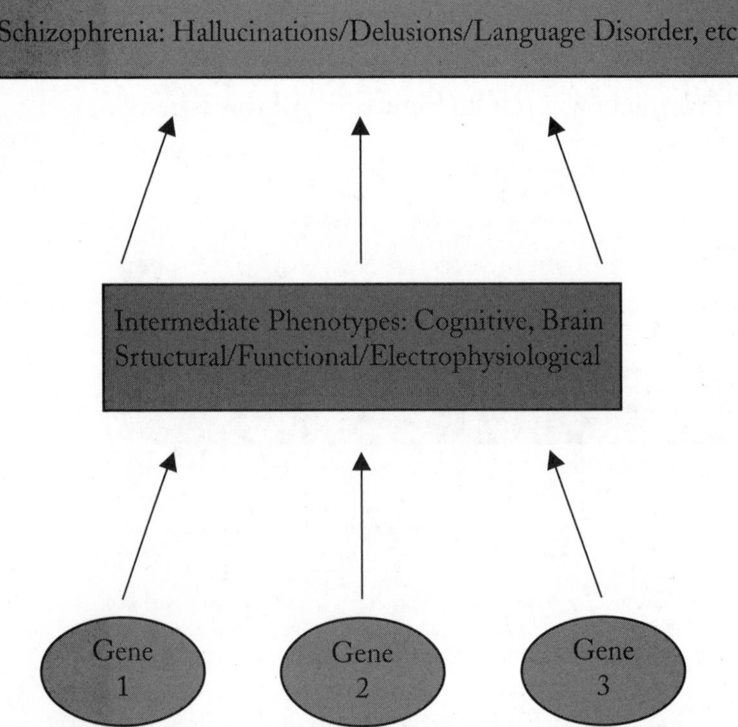

Figure 4 This diagram illustrates the "endophenotype" or intermediate phenotype concept, which is that genes do not directly cause symptoms, but rather produce something else biological that can in turn lead to the symptoms.

intermediate phenotype are that (1) the factor has to have been shown consistently to be abnormal in people who have schizophrenia compared with those who do not; (2) the factor must have been demonstrated to be inherited (i.e., runs in families); (3) within families who have inherited the factor, it should be present in all individuals who have schizophrenia; and (4) it may also be present in well family members because despite having the genes for schizophrenia, the illness does not always develop. Thus far, many brain structural changes and also changes in cognitive functioning, such as certain types of memory, have been candidates for endophenotypes, but at this time no one factor is clearly known to be intermediate between genes and the clinical manifestation of illness.

Intermediate phenotype

Sometimes also called an "endophenotype." It is the trait in genetic terms that a gene is responsible for more directly producing something else that then leads to the clinical illness itself. This is a trait that may make a person more vulnerable to getting an illness.

Phenotype

The trait that is expressed by a gene. For example, having blue eyes or brown eyes would be phenotypes. The clinical disorder called schizophrenia may also be a "phenotype" in genetic studies.

61. Will there be future DNA testing for schizophrenia?

It is highly unlikely that a specific genetic defect will be helpful for testing people to see whether they have inherited the tendency for schizophrenia. This is because, given the highly nonspecific biologic and clinical findings in schizophrenia, and given that having high-risk variants of specific genes only confers a small general risk for illness, no test will likely have enough sensitivity and specificity to be useful on a population basis for accurate testing. The one exception to this is if CNVs prove to be important findings implicating multiple rare mutations that produce disease within individual families. Thus a commercial testing for particular rare CNVs that are highly likely to be causal may be worthwhile. However, in most cases, genes established to contribute to vulnerability, will likely only be useful to provide a scientific understanding of the mechanism for schizophrenia, which can then lead to the development of new medications. Nevertheless, there are now several commercial companies that one can find on the Internet that are beginning to advertise "tests" for schizophrenia and other serious mental illnesses such as bipolar disorder. One should beware of the danger and misinterpretation of the results of these tests and not be tempted to order one. The tests are based on the very preliminary and weak genetic research findings that have been explored earlier in this book. They are not reliable indicators of who will develop schizophrenia and may only cause harm to people if they base any life decisions on what these tests show. They have little value, and there is no basis for their sale at this time and likely in the future. They are the "snake oil" of the new genetic era we find ourselves in after having had the human genome completely sequenced in laboratories.

62. Will DNA testing be useful to determine which medication to administer?

Testing to determine the best medication for a patient could be another eventual use of DNA sequence variation among individuals. Although variation in specific gene DNA may not be associated with the illness itself, the medications that suppress its symptoms may be responded to in different ways depending on the genetic makeup of each individual. For example, if some people have **enzymes** that have higher activity for inactivating a certain medication, then these people may need higher doses to get a clinical response than people with lower enzyme activity, or these individuals simply may not be responders to that particular medication. Similarly, if other individuals have low activity of an inactivating enzyme, they may have the drug in their system longer and thus be more prone to its side effects. It also may be possible in the future to predict whether someone will respond to a drug such as clozapine by

Enzymes

Proteins in the body that digest other substances through biochemical reactions. They are the "tools" of metabolism.

what alleles they carry for a specific gene. These factors, once established, could be available to clinicians so they can tailor treatment with the many available drugs to each individual's unique genetic makeup. These principles belong to the new burgeoning field of pharmacogenetics and hold promise for the future but will need several years of development to be useful.

63. Can genetic research provide new treatments?

As stated previously, an understanding of the biology of schizophrenia can only lead to better treatments, ones that can be given earlier, before pronounced clinical symptoms appear. Drug companies need what they call "targets" for drugs to act on and change, whether it is a neurochemical receptor blockade, growth of cells, activation of brain regions on an MRI scan, or a change in an EEG pattern. In turn, a change in the targets needs to be shown to be associated with improvement with a new drug. Consumers, however, need to be aware that developing drugs to targets takes a long time and is a complicated, expensive process. It takes many years for pharmaceutical companies to develop and test new drugs, and for every compound that the companies explore, many are abandoned for various reasons before they ever reach the market.

An understanding of the biology of schizophrenia can only lead to better treatments, ones that can be given earlier, before pronounced clinical symptoms appear.

64. In this new genome age, what are ethical concerns for the future?

Scientists must always take social responsibility for their discoveries. Some families are happy to know that schizophrenia has a strong genetic component because then they know that developing the illness has been out of their control and that their behavior was not responsible for making someone ill in their family.

Other families, in contrast, feel they have somehow been stigmatized and are passing on "bad blood." Scientists in collaboration with lawmakers must develop legislation that prevents the misuse of genetic data to label individuals as unfit so that these individuals will not be prevented from obtaining health insurance policies and educational and employment opportunities available to others in society based on their DNA make-up. There is also the concern that people will want genetic testing before mating to avoid raising a child who is likely to get this illness or that they will think twice about marrying someone with a family history of this illness, despite scientific knowledge that the excess genetic risk is low and not understood. You could envision numerous scenarios coming from superficial knowledge that schizophrenia is genetic.

PART FIVE

The Biology Underlying Schizophrenia: Current Research Findings

Are there any differences in the brains of people who have schizophrenia?

Should an MRI scan be performed?

Is schizophrenia a "chemical imbalance"?

More . . .

"I think you have to speculate. If I have a good idea, I tend to believe it is true. An idea is better than no idea . . . that's the way good science works. An idea can be tested, whereas if you have no idea, nothing can be tested and you don't understand anything!"

—James D. Watson in an interview published in *The New York Times*, on the 50th anniversary of the discovery of DNA (February 3, 2002)

65. *Are there any tests that can be taken from blood, urine, or spinal fluid?*

Immunoglobulins

The proteins that help the body respond to foreign substances and infections.

The answer is none at all, unlike most other biologic disease. You can find high blood sugar in diabetes or elevated **immunoglobulins** in multiple sclerosis. If only we had a good hypothesis about what to look for in schizophrenia! We always think we do for a short period of time, but then the evidence is unclear and findings "disappear." Several hypotheses have been explored over the years. Many factors were found in 24-hour urine collections, serum, and spinal fluid. The notorious "pink spot" from the 1960s to 1970s, a supposed litmus test for schizophrenia, was none other than metabolites of tea that the patients were drinking in excess. The so-called endogenous hallucinogens, chemicals produced in excess by one's own body, such as dimethyltryptamine and phenylethylamine, both turned out also to be artifactual findings, the former being caused by a laboratory method that had not been validated and the latter caused by nonspecific anxiety. Researchers have long abandoned the idea of looking for such factors; as we now know, the biology of schizophrenia is not that simple.

66. *Are there any differences in the brains of people who have schizophrenia?*

The answer to this question is yes, but in a subtle way, and no finding is specific to the illness, nor is any one finding present in all patients with schizophrenia.

Someone with schizophrenia could also have a completely normal brain. Since the beginning of the recognition of the concept of dementia praecox, Kraepelin (1907) felt that schizophrenia was a progressive brain disease. He noted in his textbook that "*the course is progressive without remissions. . . . Signs of mental deterioration may appear within a few months, and are usually well marked by the end of two years. . . . On the other hand, there are some cases. . . . which do not dement for a number of years.*" He also said early on that "in view of the clinical and anatomical facts known so far I cannot doubt we are dealing with serious . . . and only partially reversible damage to the cerebral **cortex**. . . . 75 percent of cases reach higher grades of dementia and sink deeper and deeper" (Kraepelin, 1899). By the time he published his 1919 text, he illustrated what he thought was wrong in the brain with drawings of neurons that he described as "diseased with lipoid products of disintegration." Where his notions about the brain came from, however, are unclear, as there are no careful research studies that he or anyone else published to provide evidence of these claims.

Cortex

The outer portion of the brain. It consists mostly of the "gray matter" that contains nerve cells.

Pneumoencephalography

An X-ray picture of the brain taken by injection of air into the cerebral ventricular space. Prior to the advent of CT and MRI scanning, this method was used to detect whether a patient had brain atrophy. This method is no longer in use.

By the 1930s, the technique of examining the brain by **pneumoencephalography**, a quite risky procedure of injecting air into the **ventricles** in order to observe their outline, was applied to studies of patients with schizophrenia. Many reports showed enlargement of the ventricular space in chronic schizophrenia, clearly suggestive of atrophy of the brain at an age when this should not have been present. These results went quite unnoticed by most psychiatrists in the mid-twentieth century, probably because of the rise in psychological and psychoanalytic theories and approaches to schizophrenia. When biologic psychiatry again became in vogue and new methods to examine the brain in vivo were developed, namely **computed tomography (CT)**, some exciting findings

Ventricles

As this term applies to the brain, the spaces connecting throughout the brain that provide a system for the circulation of the fluid present in the brain called cerebrospinal fluid.

Computed tomography (CT)

A form of X-ray that is able to view the brain in more detail than a standard skull X-ray.

emerged. In 1976, a very small study of severely ill patients with chronic schizophrenia was published in the medical journal *The Lancet* (Johnstone et al., 1976). It clearly showed by CT that the patients had significantly larger brain ventricular size than age-matched controls. Soon many other investigators, using much larger, more representative samples of patients, widely replicated this finding. To date, this is probably the most replicated finding in all of schizophrenia research!

Magnetic Resonance Imaging (MRI)
A method to examine the tissue of the brain using a magnetic field and computer system.

Gray matter
The brownish-gray nerve tissue of the brain and spinal cord that contains the nerve cells.

White matter
The whitish brain and spinal cord tissue composed mostly of nerve fibers and its shiny protective coat called myelin.

Superior temporal gyrus
A portion of the temporal lobe of the brain that has many functions related to language, including hearing it and speaking it.

In the late 1980s brain-imaging methods produced even better direct anatomical windows into the in vivo brain with the advent of **magnetic resonance imaging (MRI)**. The first studies, however, were performed using brain slices that were very thick, so subtle changes that occur in small brain structures or just subtle differences in general could be easily missed. Over the decade that followed, however, MRI scanning became more and more refined and brain images came to be seen in almost as much detail and contrast as direct postmortem brain visualization. MRI scanning currently is the main imaging technique used to evaluate the brains of people with schizophrenia. In MRI, the actual brain tissue, divided into the **gray matter** containing the neuronal cells and the **white matter** containing their fibrous connections, is clearly distinguishable. As a result, a number of studies have shown various differences in the brains of patients with schizophrenia. These differences mostly include volume of structures. Besides the ventricles, the volume of gray matter as a whole is significantly less, as is the size of the temporal lobe and its different subdivisions (i.e., **superior temporal gyrus** and hippocampus), frontal lobe, and corpus callosum (**Table 3** and **Figure 5**). We now know that there are also white matter changes in the fiber tracts connecting these structures.

Table 3 Brain Structures that Relate to Schizophrenia.

Brain Structure	Structure Function	Finding in Schizophrenia	Does the Finding become Greater Over Time?	Comments
Ventricles	Holds spinal fluid that bathes the brain	Enlarged	Yes	Large ventricles mean that the brain tissue surrounding it is less than it should be
Frontal lobes	• Sequential planning • Processing new memory • Speaking • Some uniquely human mentalizing	Reduced gray matter	Unknown	This structure is difficult to measure, but its functioning has been shown in many ways to be abnormal
Temporal lobes	Auditory processing	Reduced volume	Possibly for all	
Superior temporal gyrus	Language	Reduced volume		
Hippocampus	Memory	Reduced volume		

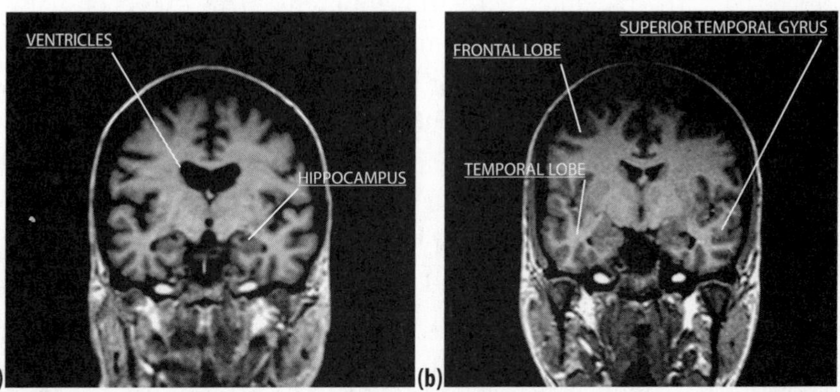

Figure 5 (a) MRI—Patient with schizophrenia. (b) MRI—Normal patient.

67. Should an MRI scan be performed?

A good evaluation of someone who is first being diagnosed with schizophrenia should include an MRI so that a baseline initial brain assessment is available for comparison in later years.

In a clinical setting, a good evaluation of someone who is first being diagnosed with schizophrenia should include an MRI so that a baseline initial brain assessment is available for comparison in later years. It should also be used to exclude any other brain diseases that could mimic the symptoms of schizophrenia, such as temporal lobe tumors, or any other known neurodegenerative disorder, no matter how rare these disorders are in people with characteristic symptoms of schizophrenia. The status of brain structural and functional findings could be helpful for considering what the likely outcome of an episode might be.

68. Are functional MRI scans useful?

Functional MRI (fMRI)
A brain scan that shows actions taking place in the brain in response to a stimulus. The stimulus could be anything, such as voluntary movement of the fingers or thinking about or distinguishing the meaning of a set of words.

Magnetic resonance spectroscopy (MRS)
A type of MRI scan that examines chemical spectras in the brain. The chemicals examined are those present in the structure of membranes or metabolic activity in nerve cells and between cells.

Some other types of MRI scans that can be performed are **functional MRI (fMRI)** or **magnetic resonance spectroscopy (MRS)**. In fMRI, subjects are given a test to perform that uses different brain anatomical regions while the scanner takes pictures of their brain. In patients with schizophrenia, the tasks usually include some type of behavior that requires a short period of memory or language detection by responding when hearing instructions or when seeing them. In general, the functioning of different parts of the brain is measurable by the intensity of activity in the working regions. Schizophrenia patients have been shown to have less focused and less lateralized functioning when responding to these tasks, although the studies thus far are just initial research findings. More needs to be done before this kind of scanning can be applied in clinical situations.

Similarly, MRS is a quantitative imaging method to detect levels of neurochemicals in the brain in different regions. Abnormal amounts of these substances are thought to indicate evidence of progressive brain disease at the biochemical level. These scans too, however, are not applicable to a clinical setting and have only been research tools that present some complicated problems thus far in their interpretation. Thus, at present, neither fMRI nor MRS are types of scans that are yet ready for the clinic. Neither are **positron emission tomography (PET) scans**, a more invasive procedure that is more useful in tumor and other neurodegenerative diseases, but not schizophrenia.

Positron emission tomography (PET) scans

A radiologic procedure that measures the metabolism of a radiolabeled substance. A substance, which is known to enter the brain relatively rapidly, is radiolabeled and then injected into a subject's bloodstream. Pictures are then taken of the brain with the regions metabolizing the injected substance "lighting up."

69. Should an EEG be done on patients with schizophrenia?

Certain findings in EEG scans are characteristic of people with schizophrenia. For example, some of the EEG brain waves that are produced when the subject is stimulated in some way are known as "evoked potentials." Patients with schizophrenia have reduced amplitudes of these waves, particularly over the frontal and temporal lobes, when they are stimulated with an odd sound or visual object. These tests might also be worth conducting because they are associated with other symptoms and, similar to the MRI, might be able to give some prognostic indication. However, for the most part, they are still considered research tools and are not available in a clinical setting. They would only be useful clinically if a seizure disorder were suspected.

70. Is schizophrenia a "chemical imbalance"?

Many people speak of schizophrenia as a "chemical imbalance," which makes sense given that the medications are chemicals that alleviate many symptoms. What this actually means, however, is still not clear in research studies, and how the chemistry interacts with the structural brain changes is not known. Many biochemical hypotheses about schizophrenia were formulated after neuroleptic medications were introduced. These drugs act directly on **dopamine** receptors, as well as other receptors, and their efficacy could be shown to be directly related specifically to dopamine activity by laboratory assays. Until recently, the dopamine hypothesis had always been the most prominent. In support of the dopamine hypothesis are studies showing that dopamine receptors measured in postmortem brain and also in PET scans were elevated in patients with schizophrenia. Some evidence showed that these findings were not due to an effect of the medication, but rather the pathology of the illness itself.

Dopamine

One of the chemical substances that is important for conveying "messages" between nerve cells in the brain.

Serotonin, another brain neurotransmitter, as well as GABA and others, has been thought to be related somehow to schizophrenia pathology, likely by its effects on dopamine receptors.

Serotonin

A hormone found in the brain, platelets, digestive tract, and pineal gland. It acts both as a neurotransmitter (a substance that nerves use to send "messages" to one another) and a vasoconstrictor (a substance that causes blood vessels to narrow). A reduction of serotonin in the brain is thought to be a cause of depression.

More recently, the "glutamate hypothesis" has become even more prominent than the dopamine hypothesis. L-glutamic acid (glutamate) is a major excitatory amino acid neurotransmitter throughout the brain and nervous system, and it is known that glutamate plays a major role in brain development, affecting neuronal migration, neuronal differentiation, axon genesis, and neuronal survival. It was first thought to be involved in schizophrenia when the popular recreational drug phencyclidine (PCP) was recognized to not only mimic schizophrenia in its actions, but also to exert its actions primarily on glutamate receptors. Several lines of evidence then suggested that a dysfunction in glutamatergic neurotransmission via the N-methyl-D-aspartate (NMDA) subtype of glutamate receptors might be involved in the pathophysiology of schizophrenia, and the NMDA receptor hypofunction hypothesis of schizophrenia became known. The dopamine hypothesis attributes hyperdopaminergic function as a possible cause of schizophrenia, whereas the glutamate hypothesis proposes a hypofunctional glutamate system. There is substantial evidence for both hypotheses, based on observations that certain classes of street drugs can produce schizophrenic-like symptoms in normal individuals. Not only does PCP produce symptoms most similar to schizophrenia by antagonizing the action of glutamate, but amphetamines also produce some of the acute positive symptoms by stimulating dopamine receptors. In general, PCP and similar drugs produce somewhat more of the symptoms of schizophrenia than the amphetamine-like drugs. The latter fail to produce some of the core symptoms of schizophrenia, such as formal thought disorder and negative symptoms, although PCP may. Currently, initiated by the glutamate hypothesis, both glycine and D-serine, NMDA receptor stimulators, are being used as add-on medications to treat patients with chronic schizophrenia who do not completely benefit from other medications.

Most recently, some pharmaceutical companies have developed new agents that target the glutamate pathway by binding to one of its receptors. Some initial trials have shown improvement in the symptoms of schizophrenia using these drugs, but more trials will need to be done before these drugs are ready for FDA approval, and toxicity will have to be carefully evaluated.

71. When do the brain changes occur, and is schizophrenia considered a progressive brain disorder?

Patients with chronic schizophrenia are known to have the changes mentioned previously that are recognized in brain structures, but at what point in a person's lifetime they begin to become abnormal is still controversial. Studies of patients at the first episode, however, are able to detect many of the changes, suggesting that they may occur early. There is some evidence from a couple of recent high-risk studies that the brain changes actually predate illness and the brain continues to deteriorate along with the development of symptoms. There is also now evidence from several studies following patients after their first episode of illness that suggests that the brain continues to change at a more rapid rate than that of the normal aging process. Brain tissue seems to be lost at a greater rate over time sporadically throughout the illness (**Figure 6**). However, while the tissue loss seems to be correlated to the severity of illness in some studies, in others it is not. It may be that a little nonsignificant tissue loss is also due to a lifetime of taking medications that affect brain functioning, but

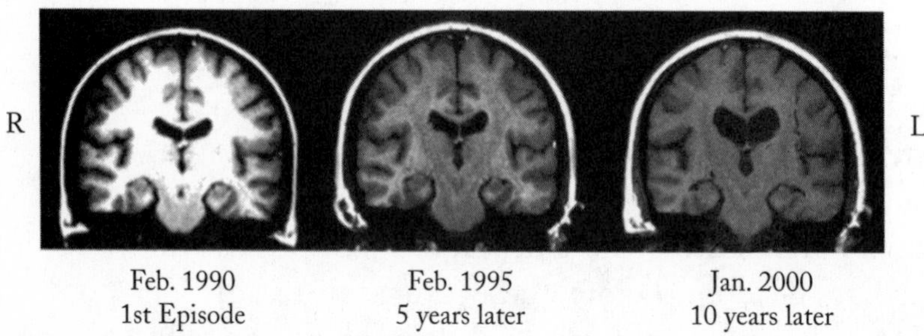

Figure 6 10-Year MRI Follow-Up. A 34-year-old female with chronic schizophrenia who has a brother with schizophrenia.

it is not clear that this is a bad thing. More research is needed on this topic, as its implications are vast. If there is progressive brain structural change characteristic of schizophrenia and it is related to the evolution of clinical symptoms, then medications need to be given early to prevent progression. Several research groups are now working on this issue and hopefully will soon produce recommendations about early treatment and the types of treatment. Table 3 in Question 66 outlines the changes that have been found in brains of patients with schizophrenia and whether there is evidence of progressive change in these structures. Figure 6 illustrates an example of one such case of a 34-year-old female with schizophrenia whose ventricles appear to have consistently enlarged over time from her first episode of illness to 5 and then 10 years later.

72. What is the neurodevelopmental hypothesis about schizophrenia?

For over a decade, most investigators have thought that the brain structural abnormalities of schizophrenia must at least in part be neurodevelopmental in origin—that is, occurring either because of an insult prenatally to the developing brain or because of a neuronal growth defect prenatally that is perhaps genetically controlled. One alternative hypothesis was that in adolescent-onset illness, the reorganization of brain connections during that time might be occurring abnormally. The reasons for constructing these theories as an alternative to thinking of schizophrenia as a progressive degenerative process mainly were that the length of illness duration could never be correlated with the amount of abnormal brain change and that no cellular signs of degeneration have ever been shown in brains of patients with schizophrenia.

It has now become clear, however, from results of carefully conducted longitudinal studies that brain ventricular size continues to expand over time and that none of the anomalies associated with schizophrenia appear static. See Figure 3 in Question 59 for a combination of both the neurodevelopmental and degenerative hypotheses.

PART SIX

Substance Abuse and Schizophrenia

Can drug use in adolescence cause schizophrenia?

Are there any specific drugs that more frequently cause schizophrenia-like symptoms?

Is it okay to drink alcohol if you have schizophrenia?

More . . .

"It was very well to say 'Drink me,' but the wise little Alice was not going to do that in a hurry. 'No, I'll look first,' she said, 'and see whether it is marked "poison" or not.' . . . However, this bottle was not marked 'poison,' so Alice ventured to taste it, and finding it very nice . . . very soon finished it off."

—Lewis Carroll, Down the Rabbit-Hole, *Alice's Adventures in Wonderland*, 1865

73. Can drug use in adolescence cause schizophrenia?

It has long been known that various street drugs are used by people who develop an acute first episode of schizophrenia and that patients and their families often blame the first episode on these drugs. Although there is an increased drug use in people developing schizophrenia compared with people of similar ages who do not use drugs, it has long been controversial as to which really comes first, drug abuse or schizophrenia. Can certain drugs cause schizophrenia, or does having subtle emotional signs of "preschizophrenia" cause people to alleviate their uncomfortable feelings or behaviors by experimenting with drugs? Some data from Europe recently indicate that in some people who are particularly frequent cannabis (marijuana) users, specifically during adolescence, the use of this substance may be causal. However, it is generally thought that because many people who use cannabis or other drugs frequently do *not* get schizophrenia, a genetic predisposition to the illness must also be present. Alternatively, the use of drugs may simply bring what is a predetermined illness on faster.

Drug use has been associated with an earlier age of onset of schizophrenia.

Drug use has been associated with an earlier age of onset of schizophrenia and with a poorer outcome and is particularly relevant to males with the illness, as males tend to abuse drugs significantly more than females.

The kind of drug that can be harmful also depends on what is popular during a particular era and what is readily available. These factors, of course, vary geographically worldwide and with time.

Various drugs that have been used and were popular at different times were also known by various street names and include amphetamines (speed or ecstasy), PCP (angel dust), lysergic acid diethylamide (LSD), and cannabis (hash, marijuana). LSD was so prevalent in the 1960s that songs were popularized about its use (e.g., "Lucy in the Sky with Diamonds" by the Beatles). LSD and PCP are considered hallucinogens in normal individuals, although other drugs have been used as such at different times, whereas cannabis in normal individuals causes a pleasant sense of well-being, and only a small portion of individuals have adverse reactions, such as hallucinatory or other scary experiences. Cannabis remains the most frequently used drug among adolescents in the United States. Unfortunately, if abused and used heavily, it has adverse consequences on the user's functioning regardless of whether it will lead to schizophrenia.

74. Can someone who has schizophrenia smoke cannabis (marijuana)?

Numerous studies now show a strong association between marijuana use and the development of schizophrenia (see Question 73). Thus, it would not be advisable for people already diagnosed with schizophrenia to use marijuana. Some believe that this newly reported association results from an increased potency in the marijuana now available on the streets, which has increased substantially over recent years. After schizophrenia is diagnosed, continued use of cannabis or marijuana, easily available compared with other street drugs, can only be harmful in causing less likelihood of response to medication. Marijuana use also initiates a lack of compliance with oral medication so that patients tend to have a poor outcome and become rehospitalized until they realize the need to stay away from marijuana. Their reactions are often not euphoric and calming as are the effects on their peers who do not have schizophrenia, although the mechanism for this difference is not known.

75. Are there any specific drugs that more frequently cause schizophrenia-like symptoms?

No street drugs are free from this association. Some of them, such as methamphetamines and PCP, are known to mimic symptoms of schizophrenia acutely in otherwise normal people who are given doses of them. Both of these drugs are epidemic in some countries. Methamphetamine use is particularly high and widely prevalent in many African countries, and thus psychiatrists in these countries are finding difficulty separating true chronic schizophrenia from continuous methamphetamine use.

76. Is it okay to drink alcohol if you have schizophrenia?

The simple answer is no. Alcohol, particularly in moderate amounts, precipitates and exacerbates the symptoms of schizophrenia as well as leads to noncompliance with a medication regime and rehospitalization in many people. It also has adverse effects on blood levels of medications and can be particularly toxic to the liver in combination with multiple drugs that are metabolized also through the liver. Consuming alcohol is certainly not advised, given that it is not easily used in careful moderation. One beer at night on a social occasion for someone with schizophrenia, however, may be beneficial if it affords a way of socializing and meeting with peers—that is, becoming more integrated into everyday life. It is the excess that is harmful to anyone, and those with schizophrenia are particularly sensitive.

77. Why do people with schizophrenia smoke cigarettes excessively?

It has long been noticed that patients on psychiatric hospital wards are almost all chain cigarette smokers, and numerous scientific surveys now confirm the association of cigarette smoking with schizophrenia. Behavioral therapies in the past were geared toward positive reinforcement by the attainment of a goal and thus winning a pack of cigarettes. You might expect lung cancer and other cigarette-associated cancers to be increased in schizophrenic patients, but this does not appear to be true.

Whether people with schizophrenia smoke cigarettes so heavily because of their underlying psychopathology or because of a social consequence of having this illness is presently unclear. It may simply be that these people develop the addictive habit of cigarette smoking because of a need to occupy their hands and stimulate themselves with some oral gratification during times that are continually stressful and uncomfortable. However, this phenomenon has been noted to have a specific scientific basis by a well-known researcher in Colorado, Dr. Robert Freedman, who claims that cigarette smoking is so excessive among these patients, namely a craving for nicotine, because of an underlying abnormality in receptors for nicotine in the brain. His laboratory, and now many others, is currently studying nicotine receptors in people with schizophrenia, the genetic susceptibility for abnormalities in these receptors, and addiction to nicotine. One possibility is that the genetic abnormality that leads to nicotine addiction may somehow be related to the genetic risk for schizophrenia. Pharmaceutical companies are thus trying to identify some novel drugs that might counteract the nicotine receptor abnormalities and thus be efficacious in alleviating symptoms of schizophrenia. However, none have yet been found.

PART SEVEN

Violence and Aggression in Schizophrenia

Do people with schizophrenia frequently commit violent acts and crimes?

What should I do if my relative or friend is behaving violently?

How can violent behavior be predicted?

"Is this a dagger I see before me,

The handle toward my hand? Come, let me clutch thee.

. . . . . .

I go, and it is done. The bell invites me.

Hear it not, Duncan; for it is a knell

That summons thee to heaven or to hell."

—Shakespeare, *Macbeth*, Act 2, Scene 1

78. Do people with schizophrenia frequently commit violent acts and crimes?

Violence is not *a symptom of schizophrenia. An individual with schizophrenia is not more dangerous than any other person, provided that he or she is treated with medication that alleviates the symptoms of this disease.*

Violence is *not* a symptom of schizophrenia. An individual with schizophrenia is not more dangerous than any other person, provided that he or she is treated with medication that alleviates the symptoms of this disease. In fact, people with schizophrenia are far more likely to harm themselves than others. However, there is a conception that people with schizophrenia are violent. This notion is likely based particularly on criminal cases that gain a lot of publicity and are subjects of movies, such as the paranoid schizophrenia patient who was released from a Long Island, New York, state psychiatric hospital many years ago, convincing his physician that he no longer had the delusion that his estranged wife must die, only to immediately go to her home and murder her, or the homeless hallucinating man who pushed a young girl onto the New York City subway track and into the path of an incoming train. Ted Kaczynski, the "Unabomber," was clearly suffering from paranoid schizophrenia and a thought disorder that was certainly evident in the manifesto he sent to *The New York Times*. In the United Kingdom, a serial killer known as the "Yorkshire Ripper," suffered from schizophrenia and was committed to a long-stay psychiatric forensic hospital after his trial. The young man with severe paranoia who shot many random people on the Long Island

Railroad certainly had all the signs of untreated paranoid schizophrenia for years, but most people did not pay enough attention to get him into treatment.

Another example, the famous young man John Hinckley, Jr., who felt the delusional need to shoot President Reagan many years ago, was diagnosed with schizophrenia and has spent many years since in a psychiatric hospital. This particular case, similar to that of the Long Island Railroad shooter, was one in which the affected individual had a long history of unstable behavior and several warning signs of psychopathological behavior that should have led family, friends, and professionals to intervene much earlier. He became over the years obsessed with the movie *Taxi Driver*, which was about an American psychopath who stalks the president of the United States. Hinckley saw himself becoming romantically involved with the actress Jodie Foster, who played an attractive young woman in the movie, and began stalking her with letters and attempted visits while she was a student at Yale. Some people say that his obsession with this movie is what drove him to purchase handguns and eventually, on March 29, 1981, to shoot and wound President Reagan and his press secretary James Brady, as well as two other individuals on the scene. He was tried and eventually found not guilty by reason of insanity and sent to the special forensic unit at St. Elizabeth's Hospital in Washington, DC. Part of the tragedy in this case is that if any of the professionals, including psychiatrists, whom Hinckley had seen during the several years preceding this event had correctly diagnosed him and treated him with neuroleptic medication, the violence he inflicted on the president and others would likely not have occurred.

Finally, most recently there is the so-called "Craigslist Killer" in Boston. The person alleged of committing this crime was a star medical student who was liked by all and not suspected of having any mental illness; yet the bizarre story of how he browsed through the erotic section of Craigslist to find women who were offering massage and other sexually provocative services is similar to the Yorkshire Ripper in many ways. Time will tell as the story unfolds whether he too was suffering from an underlying psychosis. Thus, many such stories give the public the impression that people with schizophrenia, by virtue of their diagnosis, are dangerous

Despite some of these examples, when violence does occur, it is more frequently targeted at family members and is not premeditated. Moreover, all these examples of violent crimes were committed when the perpetrator was in an unstable stage of illness that was untreated by medications or other forms of therapy mentioned in this book. The subway incident described here was the stimulus for New York State to pass a mandatory outpatient treatment law (Kendra's Law, named after the girl who was pushed onto the subway tracks and died) so that patients with schizophrenia who are released from hospitals cannot voluntarily choose to discontinue their medications. Several other states now have similar laws.

Crimes are not only acts of violence. Various other crimes, such as robbery, property damage, and many infractions of the law, can lead to jail sentences. Antisocial behavior, commonly known as psychopathy, is clearly associated with crime. Large studies of individuals with and without schizophrenia, however, do not suggest that psychopathy is associated with schizophrenia; thus, whether or not schizophrenia is present, antisocial personality disorder or psychopathy is associated with crime. In addition, family studies do not show an excess clustering of psychopathy among relatives of schizophrenic patients, indicating that this behavior is not genetically associated with schizophrenia.

79. What should I do if my relative or friend is behaving violently?

Many people close to patients with schizophrenia are frustrated with the mental healthcare system as it currently exists in the United States because in most instances it does not provide support for a sick individual until he or she is behaving dangerously toward others or acutely threatening suicide. In these circumstances, of course, the police emergency phone number (in the United States—911) should be called immediately, and the patient must be subdued and brought to a psychiatric hospital. Unfortunately, these patients are too often victims of accidental violence by frightened police who provide severe force to suppress the violent individuals, in some cases inflicting injuries and even death. Too often, patients are brought to jail and kept there for many days without much-needed medications. Police and all types of public emergency response personnel must be trained in the acute care of these individuals and how to safely transport them to psychiatric emergency rooms. Families and friends can be instrumental support at times like these to ensure that patients receive the proper treatment and legal representation.

80. How can violent behavior be predicted?

The likelihood of violence is increased by consumption of alcohol or street drugs. In addition, patients who are noncompliant with a prescribed medication regime can then become violent. The most important predictor of violent behavior is a past history of violence, whether or not someone has schizophrenia. Strong predictors of violence in the mentally ill are the feeling that others are out

The most important predictor of violent behavior is a past history of violence, whether or not someone has schizophrenia.

to harm them and the feeling that their minds are dominated by forces beyond their control or that thoughts are being put into their heads. Another symptom that may predict violence is a specific type of hallucination called "command hallucinations," in which internal voices are heard as if they were coming from the outside telling the individual what to do and in many cases to either harm oneself or someone else. The presence of this type of hallucination and the need to act on it may be a compelling predictor of violence.

Often, however, police pick up individuals with schizophrenia in general as a precautionary measure because they do not know when someone who is behaving out of the ordinary is likely to be violent. Such is especially true in Washington, DC, where caution may be essential but can sometimes be an overreaction. For example, it is common for many people with paranoid or other types of schizophrenia from all over the country to travel to the nation's capital to address their many delusions about the FBI, the Internal Revenue Service, or even the president. At St. Elizabeth's Hospital, once a federal psychiatric institution, in the late twentieth century and for many years, a special ward existed in the forensic division for the "White House cases." Anyone who threatened the president would be brought there and could not be released until the Secret Service allowed it. I once evaluated a patient on this ward whose only crime was feeling that he had many things in common with the then-president Gerald Ford and simply presented himself at the gate of the White House requesting to "share his bubble gum with President Ford"! Education of law enforcement officers, the Secret Service, and the FBI in how to predict violent behavior and also manage patients with schizophrenia is essential.

PART EIGHT

Suicidal Behavior and Schizophrenia

What are the signs of suicidal thoughts in schizophrenia?

What can be done to prevent suicide attempts?

"They heard her singing her last song,
The Lady of Shalott.
. . . . . .
Till her blood was frozen slowly,
And her eyes were darkened wholly,
. . . . . .
Who is this? And what is here?
And in the lighted palace near
Died the sound of royal cheer . . .
But Lancelot mused a little space;
He said, "She has a lovely face;
God in his mercy lend her grace,
The Lady of Shalott."

—Alfred Lord Tennyson, *The Lady of Shalott,* Part IV

For most people with schizophrenia, the most vulnerable period for suicide is when they are young, newly diagnosed, treated with medications for the first time, and then recently discharged from the hospital.

81. What are the signs of suicidal thoughts in schizophrenia?

It is commonly thought that suicide is solely a characteristic of depression, but this is not so. Approximately 1 in 10 people with schizophrenia commit suicide. The average age span of people with schizophrenia is less than that of the general population, and this may partially be due to suicide. Suicide attempts are even several-fold more common than the cases that are successfully completed.

For most people with schizophrenia, the most vulnerable period for suicide is when they are young, newly diagnosed, treated with medications for the first time, and then recently discharged from the hospital. Often these individuals have not been connected properly to supportive networks and regular treatment. They have also not been adequately educated about their illness and the need for continual medication. Frequently, they are in a state of denial so that after the symptoms have subsided, they will be back to their premorbid state and will discontinue any medication recommended. However, they find adjustment to their old lives and being able to return to the independence that they enjoyed difficult. Many friends have deserted them, and a general lack of connection and closeness exists to other people as a result. This is a period when strong support, guidance, and frequent professional observation and follow-up are needed. In addition, not being married, coming from a high socioeconomic family background, and having high intelligence and high life expectations all lead to a feeling of loss, hopelessness, and isolation. If the individual then does not comply with the prescribed treatments and turns to street drugs, the suicidal risk increases substantially.

With regard to symptoms that are likely to lead to suicide, depression, of course, is by far the most common among individuals with schizophrenia, as it is in all cases of suicide. Less frequently present are the paranoid attacks of panic that lead to suicidal acts and provide the only way out of the delusion of being chased or followed. Occasionally, patients are responding to voices commanding them to harm themselves. However, contrary to what may be generally thought, depression is actually present in the majority of people with schizophrenia at some time during the course of their illness.

In the book *Night Falls Fast*, Kay Jamison describes the development of psychotic and depressive behavior in a close friend that eventually led to suicide. Could this have been prevented if she had been there for him? This was one of her reflections that she will never be able to answer. The book, however, clearly describes all the signs of impending suicide and how one may survive them, as she herself did. Suicide is the ultimate way that people with schizophrenia deal with their struggles with thoughts and hallucinations they cannot control. These symptoms of schizophrenia cause pain as clearly as physical injuries can. Individuals with this disorder may eventually commit suicide because of the "pain," hence the subtitle of this book, "*Painful Minds*."

82. What can be done to prevent suicide attempts?

The foremost important preventive measure is to provide intensive frequent follow-up for newly diagnosed patients. Support systems must be in place before release of such patients from the hospital, and these must include not only psychiatric care but also occupational rehabilitation, family support, social support, financial support, and, finally, follow-up by healthcare personnel to make sure that a comprehensive treatment plan occurs.

It is now thought that certain medications may be particularly beneficial and protective against suicidal thoughts, although the mechanism for this action is not clearly understood. One such medication that has been shown in a large trial to lead to significantly less suicidal behavior than other medications is clozapine. This effect may be due to clozapine's prominent stimulant action on serotonin receptors in the brain, although this is only a theory. Suicide has long been associated with low brain levels of the metabolites of serotonin and may indicate low serotonergic tone in the brain. Serotonin is a neurotransmitter that is abundant in brain regions that are associated with emotion. It is thus possible that low moods are a reflection of low serotonin, which is supported by the knowledge that newer antidepressants called the selective serotonin reuptake inhibitors (SSRIs) raise the availability of serotonin in brain tissue and are helpful in alleviating depression, whether or not depression is the primary diagnosis.

PART NINE

Issues for Women

Is schizophrenia different in women?

Should patients who are pregnant take medication for schizophrenia?

What is the risk of a postpartum relapse?

More . . .

"The day will come when man will recognize woman as his peer, not only at the fireside, but in councils of the nation. Then, and not until then, will there be a perfect comradeship, the ideal union between the sexes that will result in the highest development of the race."

—Susan B. Anthony

"Remember, no one can make you feel inferior without your consent."

—Eleanor Roosevelt

"Tell us what it is to be a woman so that we may know what it is to be a man."

—Toni Morrison, Nobel Lecture, 1993

83. Is schizophrenia different in women?

For many years in the United States and elsewhere, women were placed in psychiatric hospitals for long periods of time and institutionalized simply for having a domineering husband and dysfunctional family life. Husbands who wished to discard their wives could sign commitment papers and claim psychiatric symptoms in their wives in order to do so. Geller and Harris (1994) have documented such treatment of women from as early as 1840 through 1945. More humane treatment and legislation against involuntary hospitalization for less than acutely dangerous conditions have abolished these inequities, but they remain documented in the history of psychiatry.

In fact, there is no reason to keep many women hospitalized for long periods of time, as schizophrenia has a much better outcome in women than men overall. Women have a later age of onset than men on average and may also have a different cluster of symptoms, and they are more likely to have a brief psychotic episode that resolves more quickly than men. Women also are less aggressive than men when unmedicated, are not prone to committing violent acts as frequently, and thus are not a danger to other people. The poorer social outcome for men than women can be attributed to not having reached as high a level of social development by the time of onset than women. Thus, age at onset of the biology of schizophrenia may be the key variable.

Late-onset schizophrenia (i.e., onset after the age of 40 years) is almost exclusively in women. Women are more often diagnosed with schizoaffective disorder and less likely with paranoid schizophrenia than men, but how much of this difference might be cultural, at least in part, is unknown. Pharmacotherapy in women should also be different because the response of women to medications may differ from that of men. They require lower doses in order to suppress symptoms, and some serious side effects are more often seen in women than men. Drug trials, however, specifically comparing women with men that are controlled for various environmental and other factors that could affect drug levels and thus treatment response (such as cigarette smoking) are far too few. Women tend to be ignored and even eliminated from research clinical trials.

A common notion to explain sex differences is that **estrogen** levels must have a protective effect on the development of schizophrenia. Studies show a modulation of the dopamine D_2 receptors by estrogen and also that estrogen in some studies has a weak neuroleptic-like effect. This effect is not the only explanation for sex differences, however. In fact, genetics also clearly plays a role in actual age of onset. Despite the age of onset for schizophrenia being on average a couple of years later in women than men, when more than one individual within a family has schizophrenia, the age of onset tends to be highly similar regardless of the sex of

Estrogen

A female hormone that is produced in the female organs (ovaries). It is produced in different amounts throughout the menstrual cycle and is reduced after menopause.

the affected individuals. This implies that inheritance also influences the age of onset. If the sex differences in schizophrenia are genetic, then a gene that at least modifies the illness expression, or even causes it entirely, may be on the sex chromosomes. Although this theory has not yet been proven, it is currently openly debated (DeLisi & Crow, 1989).

84. Should patients who are pregnant take medication for schizophrenia?

Women who take antipsychotic medication, because of the hyperprolactinemia it causes, are less fertile than women who are not on these medications. Exposing the developing infant prenatally or through lactation to antipsychotic medication could also have long-term sequelae. There is an increased risk for congenital malformations in offspring of mothers who were administered neuroleptics during pregnancy, particularly during the earlier weeks of pregnancy (weeks 4 through 10), and we have little data on the effects of the newer atypical medications.

The establishment of recommended dosing for women during pregnancy has not been adequately studied, nor has any treatment trial been performed comparing different neuroleptic treatments for their subsequent effect on the developing fetus. The lack of this research is unwarranted, but even to date, it goes unnoticed. The excuse of many researchers usually is that hormonal changes cannot be controlled in research studies, thus making interpretation of any study results on women difficult. It also may be, however, that the hormonal modification of the action of some neuroleptics may allow for lower doses to be given during pregnancy, but this needs to be carefully examined. The pharmacologic management of women in the perinatal period when hormonal status suddenly changes is also very important, and little has been described about this condition in the literature.

Having schizophrenia also leads to an increased risk for obstetrical complications, including preterm deliveries and a low-birth-weight infant. The influence of maternal intake of neuroleptics, and also the stability of the mother's psychiatric condition on the development of obstetric complications is unknown. In general, women with schizophrenia tend to receive poorer prenatal medical care, and this too may lead to complications as a consequence. It is clear that not enough research has been done on pregnancy in schizophrenia. Overall, the risk of withholding medication to suppress psychosis must be weighed against the risk to the fetus and to the mother.

In addition, women with schizophrenia have higher rates of forced sex and unwanted pregnancies. They may also have a reduced capacity to provide mothering and to respond to their child's needs and thus require special guidance to overcome and deal with these circumstances and deficits.

85. What is the risk of a postpartum relapse?

Special support after birth for women with schizophrenia needs to be intensive and postpartum relapse prevented or detected early so that treatment can quickly be augmented. The risk of a postpartum psychiatric disorder, particularly depression and psychosis, is higher in women with a prior psychiatric history than in those without it. The change in hormone levels during the perinatal period may also warrant change in neuroleptic dose.

The risk of a postpartum psychiatric disorder, particularly depression and psychosis, is higher in women with a prior psychiatric history than in those without it.

Unfortunately, there have been too many highly publicized cases in the United States of mothers who either have a postpartum relapse of their illness or have a first episode of a psychosis during the postpartum period as long as 6 months after giving birth. At the extreme, these women can be very harmful to their children and have been known to kill them because of various delusional beliefs, such as in the famous Andrea Yates case. Yates had multiple delusions about her children being cursed by the devil, and she acted upon her need to supposedly end their suffering by drowning them one by one. Her husband was remarkably unaware that she had psychiatric problems and failed to pick up on any warning signs. Such tragic events could be avoided with careful recognition and treatment of high-risk postpartum women by healthcare professionals and the education of close family members.

86. What about breast-feeding?

Postpartum lactation and breast-feeding may augment the higher prolactin levels already present during conventional antipsychotic treatment. Breast milk, however, likely excretes neuroleptics, and thus breast-feeding should be cautioned against in medicated patients. We do not know the effect of neuroleptics on the developing infant but assume there could be lasting effects on the brain and nervous system. There are no studies of children of breast-feeding patients on neuroleptics, nor are there studies of the new atypical neuroleptics to see whether they are safer than old-generation neuroleptics for women. It is presently unknown whether any of these medications, including antidepressants, affect brain growth and development, although it is now known that the SSRIs can increase brain-derived neurotrophic factor (BDNF) and thus may have some effect, beneficial or not, on the developing brain. Nevertheless, it is recommended that women on these medications do not breast-feed their children. It is hoped that the pharmaceutical industry will take the responsibility to investigate these important issues in the near future.

87. Can estrogen for birth control help suppress symptoms?

Often women who have schizophrenia and are sexually active do not use contraceptives and frequently are not compliant with oral contraceptives; thus, if warranted, the use of long-acting contraceptive medications is the method of choice. Whether these treatments augment the effects of antipsychotic medication has been little studied. Although there have been studies to suggest this interaction, as mentioned previously, large-scale studies of women have not been a focus in research studies. It is also of interest that drug trials of the new antipsychotics that do include women do not take into account whether women are administered oral contraceptives. Again, systematic trials need to be supported by the pharmaceutical companies because a few small studies suggest an augmenting antipsychotic effect of estrogen in women.

PART TEN

The Homeless and Schizophrenia

How prevalent is schizophrenia among the homeless?

What causes homelessness?

Can homeless people be forced into shelters and hospitals?

"There was a table set out under the tree . . . and the March Hare and the Hatter were having tea at it: a Dormouse was sitting between them, fast asleep, and the other two were using it as a cushion, resting their elbows on it, and talking over its head. 'Very uncomfortable for the Dormouse,' thought Alice, 'only, as it's asleep, I suppose it doesn't mind.'"

—Lewis Carroll, *Alice's Adventures in Wonderland,* 1865

88. How prevalent is schizophrenia among the homeless?

Many of us walk, or jump, over homeless men and women dressed in multiple layers of old clothes and sleeping on city sidewalk-heated grates, not possibly understanding how they could feel and rationalizing that their sleeping souls are oblivious to the cold and pain. The argument given by some is that they prefer living that way and if given housing would choose not to take it. Do we know, however, whether those that are homeless have the capacity to make this decision? Recent research surveys indicate that many of the urban homeless would be diagnosed with schizophrenia. One such patient of mine was homeless in the winter and was said to have chosen to be. He was found very cold one day and brought to a hospital nonresponsive and lost both legs below the knees due to frostbite and almost died. Perhaps *because* of their illness these individuals are incapable of seeking shelter.

Recent research surveys indicate that many of the urban homeless would be diagnosed with schizophrenia. One such patient of mine was homeless in the winter and was said to have chosen to be.

Historically, before the rise of public mental institutions run by the states, it was widely known that a high percentage of the homeless individuals lining urban streets had mental illness. It was, in fact, in part for this very reason that psychiatric institutions came into existence in large numbers (detailed in Torrey, 1988). However, the community mental health center concept that was promoted in the 1960s, combined with the wide-scale use of neuroleptic medication in public psychiatric hospitals, produced a movement for reintegrating these institutionalized people with schizophrenia back into the community. This program, provided for by funds from the federal government in the United States, and similar such projects in other countries, established outpatient mental health centers within local communities. These local centers largely failed, however. Primarily, there were not enough community care homes with adequate facilities for patients to be moved to, and the funds provided were inadequate to keep the centers and the corresponding residential facilities maintained. Thus, this so-called worldwide deinstitutionalization came full-circle again to massive increases in homelessness.

Another problem was the lack of coordination of the inpatient care with referral systems to the community mental health centers. Thus, the centers treated many more mildly ill patients who were never before in need of hospitalization, whereas those who were released from the psychiatric hospitals had difficulty becoming integrated into the healthcare system. These newly released patients would then not continue their medication and lose the ability to care for themselves and to plan daily living and coping strategies, and so they took to the streets.

Among homeless women in one study, the prevalence of psychiatric disorders was 71%, with substance abuse the leading disorder (43%), followed by anxiety disorders (35%), and then schizophrenia (12%). Many other studies find similar rates for schizophrenia among the homeless ranging from ranging from 2% to 45% internationally and with an average of 11% worldwide, with rates somewhat higher in women than men and higher in the young and the chronically homeless. Suicide rates are also higher in the homeless in general than non-homeless, regardless of psychiatric diagnosis.

Homelessness: Programs and the People They Serve, is a set of publications and a collaborative effort of the Census Bureau and the U.S. Department of Housing and Urban Development. Using statistics from 1996, the study's findings are eye opening at the very least. Of the homeless individuals surveyed, 38% report evidence of alcohol use problems in the past month, 28% report drug use problems, 39% report some evidence of mental health problems, and 66% report indicators of one or more of these problems. Information about what homelessness is and what is being done about it is available from the following sources:

- U.S. Department of Housing and Urban Development's Office of Policy Development and Research
  Phone: 1-800-245-2691
  Web site: www.hud.gov/offices/cpd/homeless/
- National Alliance to End Homelessness
  Address: 1518 K Street NW, Suite 206,
  Washington, DC 20005
  Phone: 1-202-638-1526
  E-mail: naeh@naeh.org
  Web site: www.endhomelessness.org/

89. What causes homelessness?

On a general level, homelessness is caused by poverty and unemployment, but how a person gets to that extreme level and makes the choice to give up and live on the street is more complex. People living at or below the federal poverty level are the most vulnerable to experiencing a homeless episode. The estimated annual projections account for 6.3% to 9.6% of the total U.S.

population in poverty and 6.2% to 9.3% of children in poverty. Estimates show that worldwide at least 1.3 million people are homeless—that is, without even basic minimal shelter. Even in a booming economy, at least 2.3 million adults and children, or nearly 1% of the U.S. population, are likely to experience a spell of homelessness at least once during a year. In 2009, reflecting an economic recession worldwide, the statistics grew even higher, with higher unemployment rates and a failed credit market for homes. Fleeing from violence was a predominant reason for women to be homeless, which differed markedly from male homelessness. Homelessness in people with schizophrenia has been blamed on a failure of the mental health system to provide adequate care for patients after they are discharged from the hospital. There continues to exist, however, the possibility that the nature of schizophrenia itself and its negative symptoms create homelessness, not for economic reasons, but because these people fail to use cognitive planning abilities to provide themselves with proper shelter, a very basic aspect of human survival.

90. Can homeless people be forced into shelters and hospitals?

Interestingly, a decade or more ago, many more homeless people were on the streets of New York City. What reduced this number so drastically? It was not the better treatment of patients with schizophrenia and/or drug abuse in psychiatric facilities, but it was rather the leadership of the then mayor of New York, Rudi Giuliani. His goal was to move all of the homeless off the streets and from public parks; although new shelters were built, this goal was mainly realized by using police to force the homeless off the streets and off of park benches at night, placing them mostly in jails when they did not go to shelters. If homeless individuals are not acutely harmful to themselves or others, they cannot be forced into psychiatric treatment and medication. They can, however, be picked up for "loitering" or other crimes and be placed in jail. Often, mentally ill persons confined to jail unfortunately do not receive proper medical treatment.

Homelessness remains one of America's most complicated and important social issues. Chronic poverty, coupled with physical and other disabilities, has combined with rapid changes in society, the workplace, and local housing markets to make many people vulnerable to becoming homeless. With the enactment of the Stewart B. McKinney Homeless Assistance Act of 1987, Congress recognized the need to supplement "mainstream" federally funded housing and human services programs with funding that was specifically targeted to assist homeless people. The program that was established includes provisions for emergency shelters, transitional housing programs, permanent housing programs for formerly homeless people, programs distributing vouchers for emergency accommodation, housing facilities accepting vouchers in exchange for emergency accommodation, food pantries, soup kitchens, mobile food programs, physical healthcare programs, mental healthcare programs, alcohol/drug programs, HIV/AIDS programs, outreach programs, drop-in centers, and temporary "camps" that provide emergency shelter for homeless people who seek temporary farming jobs from one state to another (the so-called "migrant workers").

Thus, over the past decade, there has been tremendous growth in services for the homeless. The shelter and housing capacity in the United States within the homeless assistance network grew by 220% between

1988 and 1996, from 275,000 beds to almost 608,000 beds in 1996. Much of the growth is due to new funding and to priorities placed on developing transitional and permanent housing programs for these people. Between 1988 and 1996, the number of such units grew from close to 0 to about 274,000 compared with the capacity of emergency shelters, which grew by only 21%. Soup kitchen and meal distribution services in central cities nearly quadrupled between 1987 and 1996, from 97,000 to 382,100 meals on an average day in winter 1996. Nationally, these programs expected to serve almost 570,000 meals, approximately one-third of which were served outside of central cities. Other types of homeless services have also increased, including outreach programs, and drop-in health centers.

PART ELEVEN

Living with Schizophrenia

Can a person with schizophrenia be professionally creative?

Should I adopt a baby whose birth parent had schizophrenia?

Should a person with schizophrenia drive a car?

More . . .

"Whatever meaning people feel can be derived from their personal suffering, to live without pain would, I believe, be even more meaningful, even more human."

—Deepak Chopra, *Unconditional Life: Discovering the Power to Fulfill Your Dreams*, 1991

91. What are the origins of the stigma attached to having schizophrenia?

Stigma

Literally a "mark"; something visible to others that sets an individual apart from others whether for justified or unjustified reasons.

The word **stigma** dates back to the ancient Greeks who defined it as something unusual about someone's body that suggests something bad and immoral. This term is widely used synonymously with something disgraceful or that of which to be ashamed. In general, a stigmatizing trait is one that turns people away from an individual, as it is assumed that this person is less than human. Anyone who does not behave within the norms accepted by "society" is stigmatized in a similar manner to minority racial stigmatization.

For many decades, families who had affected psychotic individuals would hide them in attics, closets, and basements; this was more easily done in rural than urban settings. There was the fear of a family being stigmatized if one of its members had a mental illness. Until recently, having depression was similar. Over the last decade, however, when individuals who are well respected in the community have gone public with their illnesses (such as Kay Jamison, Mike Wallace, Margot Kidder, Brian Wilson, and others) and published books on the topic, awareness that depression and bipolar disorder are diseases that can be treated has slowly taken place. People with these illnesses may still be stigmatized, but less so than in the past. Public education and awareness have helped to reduce the stigma.

This social acceptance has been less so for schizophrenia, probably because people with this illness do not make good advocates for themselves. Their prominent language and thought disorders, along with residual negative symptoms, as well as some cognitive impairment, prevent them from speaking out and becoming proactive. Thus, it has been up to their families to form public advocacy groups. The many support groups having members coming from well-respected families in the community have helped to establish public networks for regular meeting and education and to lobby for the rights of the disabled mentally ill. With new medications and the return of people with schizophrenia to productive lives, and with the knowledge that these are not people to be feared, stigma can be reduced.

With new medications and the return of people with schizophrenia to productive lives, and with the knowledge that these are not people to be feared, stigma can be reduced.

92. Can a person with schizophrenia be professionally creative?

Many examples of famous creative people with schizophrenia are available, such as John Nash who received the Nobel Prize for his work on game theory, the artist Van Gogh, or several musicians. Creativity is usually more frequently associated with manic-depressive psychosis (bipolarity) than schizophrenia because in mania there is a flurry of grandiose thoughts and an excess of energy, whereas in schizophrenia, there is withdrawal and a loss of internal drive as well as disorganization of thoughts. It is usually the exceptional person (such as John Nash) who was highly creative prior to having full-blown schizophrenia, that is still able to retain some semblance of that level of functioning even after the chronic illness sets in. However, this person never fully returns to that level of fully creative intellectually productive state again. John Nash is famous for what he accomplished at a young age before the onset of his psychosis; he was never as productive as he would have been had he not developed schizophrenia, although he remained for many years on the Princeton campus able to inspire students to be productive in the field of mathematics.

93. Should I adopt a baby whose birth parent had schizophrenia?

There is a 10-fold, or slightly less, increase in risk over the general population for a child to develop schizophrenia when a parent has been affected. Thus, adoption of such a child should be treated with caution. The child may appear normal for many years but then tragically become ill after many years of devotion from adoptive parents. The decision is personal but should be considered seriously, at least until medications become available that can be administered early on to prevent a full-blown illness (see Part 4 on genetic risk). Adoption agencies should at least now inform prospective families of this history, and, if not, the prospective parents should request the information. We now know much more about the genetics of diseases once not recognized as inherited or biologic. It may be useful to consult either a research psychiatrist who specializes in genetic studies or a genetic counselor who is trained in these issues. While it is highly unlikely that genetic testing will be useful for schizophrenia, other diseases at least may be ruled out by genetic testing, such as Huntington's chorea or phenylketonuria, and thus before adoption, this could be warranted.

94. Should a person with schizophrenia drive a car?

Losing one's driver's license or having to forfeit the ability to drive is a loss of independence that is very difficult for anyone to adjust to, and not any less so for people with schizophrenia. However, for the safety of others on the road, others will have to firmly remove his or her permission to drive. This should be on an individual basis, particularly for a patient who is either unreliably taking medications or whose symptoms never fully abate. For example, I had a patient who entered the hospital after the last of a series of car accidents, having run a red light because he became unusually frightened seeing a police car in his rear-view window when he stopped at an intersection. His baseline paranoia had gotten the best of him and he rammed into another car; luckily no one was injured. Yet his family did not want to take the steps of having his license removed. It was I who had to inform authorities that this person should not have the privilege of being on the road.

"Road rage" has become a problem on some city highways, particularly when traffic is heavy and people do not have the patience to wait their turn or deal with the driver next to them who is not keeping up with traffic. If someone has a mental illness, particularly with paranoid and irritable traits, it may be difficult to deal with such other drivers, either because suspicion about these other drivers can quickly become manifest or because the stress of driving in general cannot be dealt with. Thus, these concerns also must be taken into account when considering the readiness for driving of someone recovering from a schizophrenia episode.

As reaction time tests and simulated driving studies have shown, people with schizophrenia tend not to be able to respond as quickly in a coordinated manner to unexpected changes in driving conditions. Although there are no known statistics on the rates of accidents in people with schizophrenia, you would expect that it could be significantly higher for people with schizophrenia than in the general population.

Nevertheless, some statistics show that 50% of outpatients with schizophrenia drive automobiles. Antipsychotic medication can affect the ability to drive, although some indication exists that atypical antipsychotics may not have this effect. However, providing that a person is not on a sedating medication that causes drowsiness and thus affects driving response, patients with schizophrenia who have been stabilized and are not preoccupied with unsuppressed symptoms are likely responsible drivers on roads that are uncomplicated, short distances, and generally not abnormally stressful driving stretches. Under no circumstances should a patient drive when he or she is experiencing an acute episode that is not stabilized with medication.

Whether a patient should drive an automobile should be considered on an individual basis. In the future, state driving tests may be modified so that all individuals might be required to take a stimulus-response test. Certainly other medical conditions, such as substance abuse, aging, and other neurological diseases, can hamper driving ability, as well as the newer problem of addiction to cell phones and text messaging while driving in otherwise normal individuals. Schizophrenia should not be singled out.

PART TWELVE

Ethical Issues

What does "involuntary" hospital commitment involve?

What is the legal insanity defense?

Do patients with schizophrenia have the capacity to give informed consent for research and other procedures?

More . . .

"They have said that he was like George Washington and his only crime was his unswerving and uncompromising patriotism, that he was not guilty of treason, that he was not a Fascist, that he was not anti-Semitic, that he was deprived of his rights to a fair trial, and that he was held as a political prisoner. The biggest myth, however, was that he was insane."

—E. Fuller Torrey, on beginning his book about Ezra Pound's psychiatric hospitalization, 1984

"The Hadamar gas chamber was set up in the basement. . . . At the conclusion of the admission procedures the nurse would tell the patients they were to have a nice shower. . . . The unsuspecting patients would have no objection to such a suggestion . . . and the director of the Hadamar center presided over a cocktail party commemorating the killing of their ten-thousandth patient."

—Hugh Gregory Gallagher, *By Trust Betrayed*, 1995

95. What does "involuntary" hospital commitment involve?

Many years ago a disgruntled husband could put away his wife for years in a psychiatric hospital. Now, however, there are laws to prevent this. Although the rules of each state and each country vary, in general, when individuals are acutely ill and unable to understand what is happening in order to make personal decisions and when they are considered a danger to themselves or others, they can be held involuntarily in psychiatric hospitalized treatment for a short period of time, renewable by two physicians. Court hearings can also resolve disputes if the patients continue to request hospital discharge but the doctors advise otherwise.

Sometimes outpatient commitment is also made mandatory so that patients are required to continue medication even when they do not have insight into the fact that they are ill and in need of the long-term medications. In this case, the only way they would be allowed by law to stay out of the hospital and in the community is if they comply with the court-ordered medication. Sometimes the law can be on the side of the patient who might still be harmful and manage to conceal this behavior. If patients are rational and fail to admit their intentions, there is no way of keeping them in the hospital confined against their will, as was the case with the patient from Long Island who was able to conceal his pathological wish to kill his wife from doctors and nursing staff and left the grounds of Pilgrim State Hospital on a day pass, shortly afterward only to murder his wife.

A related issue is whether a psychiatrist has the responsibility to divulge information received during the doctor–patient relationship if it could imply harm toward another person. One legal issue, known as the Tarasoff case, arose in California in the mid-1970s. A patient informed his doctor that he felt like harming his wife. Although the doctor called the police, who were not psychiatrically trained and thus did nothing, he failed to warn the intended victim, who was indeed murdered by the patient. This court ruling made it the responsibility of a doctor to warn an intended victim about possible harm. In another case in North Carolina, a psychiatrist was held responsible for a former patient's murderous spree 8 months after he was no longer in the psychiatrist's care. A jury found the psychiatrist culpable because when he last saw the patient, the doctor did not follow through to make sure his recommendations for seeking further care and continuing medications were adhered to. Many states now have legal ways to go around the patient-doctor confidentiality rule with record documentation that patients have been told that any information they give to a doctor may be given to others as needed, such as to a judge in court.

Nevertheless, patients who have been hospitalized in USA state institutions, Veterans Administration, or other public hospital locked wards are often there for months. Most have not committed the kind of crimes mentioned earlier but are confined in what often feels like jail. As patients become stable, the ward staff must then decide whether they are capable of having privileges to be free to walk on the grounds of the hospital or even go on passes into the nearby town. These decisions are often difficult, and care is taken when making them, weighing the patients' ability to conduct themselves responsibly and not be harmful to themselves or others.

96. What is the legal insanity defense?

An insanity defense is a legal term that excuses people with mental illness from legal responsibility for their crime. Many jurisdictions allow insanity defenses to be entered on behalf of an offender even when the defendant objects. By far the most frequent psychiatric condition associated with an insanity defense is schizophrenia. Psychiatrists in forming professional opinions about a particular case may need to change their views depending on the actual legal definition, as defined by each jurisdiction. Psychiatrists are not accustomed to these legal terms. Someone can be acutely psychotic but still able to understand the difference between right and wrong actions. Or, someone may commit a criminal act without understanding his or her actions (e.g., the man who kills his grandparents because "voices" told him to do it and because he "knew" that they were about to kill him, or the woman who drove her children into a lake, drowning them). The question becomes whether or not the individual knowingly did something wrong. Did the man commit a crime who drove his car through the White House gates because he thought it was the only way to let the president know his opinions?

By far the most frequent psychiatric condition associated with an insanity defense is schizophrenia.

Finally, with respect to the release of those people who have committed a crime and gone to mental hospitals rather than jail, in New York the Insanity Defense Reform Act was passed in 1980 and specified the procedures necessary for releasing persons to the community who were found not guilty of a criminal offense by reason of insanity. The most important condition was participation in an outpatient treatment program. Some follow-up studies, however, have found that one-fourth to one-third of these patients were rearrested, many for crimes of violence, and others were rehospitalized and their releases revoked. These people obviously constitute a special group of patients who upon hospital release need long-term treatment and social guidance in the community with close follow-up.

In some countries, such as Cuba during the 1970s and Ireland in the 1800s, as well as other parts of the United Kingdom, the criminally insane were released but were deported to other countries. Although this obviously does not solve the problem for the patients, the country of origin feels healthier.

Interestingly, some surveys actually show that those with psychotic diagnoses, such as schizophrenia, tend to be most of the criminals who obtain insanity defenses, whereas those with a prior criminal history, personality disorders, or drug and alcohol charges tend not to enter insanity pleas. Also, there is still a racial disparity so that whites are more likely to be successful with an insanity defense than people from minority backgrounds in the United States. Some thought should be given to such biases.

97. Have there been abuses of the insanity defense?

Many states would like to eliminate the insanity defense because medication may not cure some criminal behavior.

After having murdered, a person may not hesitate to do it again. Certainly, John Hinckley, who is on medication and is still in St. Elizabeth's Hospital for having shot President Reagan and stalked a movie star, no longer has the delusions that led him there; nevertheless, aside from home visits, he has never been allowed discharge and will likely live his entire life in the hospital because of the publicity associated with his case and the nature of his delusions in regard to national political interests.

There have, on the other hand, been historical political abuses of psychiatric diagnoses and the need for hospitalization. During the late 1970s, the World Psychiatric Association was investigating Russian psychiatrists for the hospitalization of political dissidents under the guise of having a particular form of politically invented schizophrenia. More recently, the same practices have been suggested to be taking place in China. Some people have suggested that when Ezra Pound, the poet, was hospitalized at St. Elizabeth's in Washington, DC, for many years, it was because of his extreme anti-American political views—not because he was psychotic. The 2009 movie *Changeling,* nominated for an Academy Award, depicts the corrupt practice in the 1920s of hospitalizing in psychiatric inpatient units people who did not comply with Los Angeles police actions. In this movie, a young mother whose child had disappeared and who pestered the police to continue searching for him was placed on a psychiatric ward, told she was delusional, and given ECT.

Patient abuses certainly exist as well. Someone who commits a crime can also be astute enough to know that an insanity defense might mean confinement in a psychiatric hospital until the psychiatric condition resolves and then freedom. Thus, symptoms can be mimicked and then resolved. The dilemma is that the only way one can diagnose schizophrenia is by the patient's admission of symptoms and observation of his or her behavior. Sometimes a distinction between malingering and the real illness cannot be ascertained; however, by interviewing a relative or close friend who has observed the patient over time and at other occasions, a more comprehensive picture of the person emerges.

The other side to this issue is that people with mental illness are often placed in prison instead of a psychiatric hospital and then are likely not to receive the treatment they need for their illness. Frequently they have no insight into their illness, and they deny symptoms when prodded. It is only the astute psychiatrist who can properly diagnose an inmate in this situation. The following excerpt from *The New York Times* provides an example of the currently existing problems in prisons when it comes to the management of people with serious mental illness (February 28, 2005):

"In City's Jails, Missed Signals Open Way to Season of Suicides," by Paul von Zielbauer

Prison Health Services and New York City's correction system share the blame for a spate of inmate suicides in 2003, government investigators said. . . . The New York Times' *year-long examination of Prison Health Services, the biggest commercial provider of medical care to inmates, found instances of disturbing deaths and other troubling treatment. The warnings were right there in her medical file: a childhood of sexual abuse, a diagnosis of manic depression, a suicide attempt at age 13—all noted when Carina Montes arrived at Rikers Island in September 2002. State investigators said that none of them were ever seen by the mental health specialist caring for her. He could never track down the file, which by December included another troubling fact: Ms. Montes had been placed on suicide watch by a jail social worker. Not that the suicide watch was terribly reliable; it depended in part on inmates paid 39 cents an hour to check on their suicidal peers. In her 5 months at Rikers, investigators later discovered that Ms. Montes never saw a psychiatrist.*

It did not, however, take a psychiatrist to pick up on the alarms she sounded near the end, when another inmate saw her tearing bed sheets and threatening to kill herself. But the guard who was called had no idea she was on suicide watch, did not notice the sheets and never reported the incident. Six hours later Ms. Montes was dead, hanging from a sheet tied to a ventilation grate. She was 29. Her offense: shoplifting 30 lipsticks. The death of Carina Montes was one in a spate of suicides in New York City jails in 2003—six in just 6 months, more than in any similar stretch since 1985. None of these people had been convicted of the charges that put them in jail. But in Ms. Montes's death and four of the five others, government investigators reached a stinging judgment about one or both of the authorities responsible for their safety: Prison Health Services, the nation's largest for-profit provider of inmate medical care, and the city correction system. In their reports, investigators faulted a system in which patients' charts were missing, alerts about despondent inmates were lost or unheeded, and neither medical personnel nor correction officers were properly trained in preventing suicide, the leading cause of deaths in American jails.

98. Do patients with schizophrenia have the capacity to give informed consent for research and other procedures?

Stabilized chronic patients with schizophrenia who are currently functioning outside of a hospital in a group home or independently almost always have the capacity to understand the information that is being presented. The question has remained about those who are incapable of living outside of the hospital, who are in a supervised environment, or who are experiencing an acute psychotic episode. In general, people with schizophrenia still have the capacity to understand instructions if things are explained clearly and slowly, and they are given the opportunity to ask questions. They also have decisional capacity and the ability to exercise their will voluntarily if the time is taken to explain information. Their attention span and preoccupation with their thought disorders and hallucinations during an acute episode makes them appear not to understand. To obtain such evidence of capacity, patients can be explained things carefully and then asked questions to see whether they understood. Also, structured capacity tests can be given to each patient. There is great sensitivity now among legislatures, academicians, researchers, and institutional review boards for human research, and careful rules must be followed to obtain written informed consent from subjects for all kinds of research studies. People who have diseases that reduce their capacity to understand what they are participating in, depending on the nature of a study or procedure, can have legal guardians give consent for them. They may also need a legal guardian to take care of their everyday affairs, particularly finances.

In general, people with schizophrenia still have the capacity to understand instructions if things are explained clearly and slowly, and they are given the opportunity to ask questions.

With respect to research participation, progress aimed toward finding better treatments for these disorders is essential; thus, alternative provisions, such as the ability to have a legal guardian to consent who can weigh the risks and benefits carefully, are important. Unfortunately, our country, as well as others, has in its too-recent history evidence of abuses by researchers of groups of people who cannot protect their individual rights, such as those who are mentally retarded or demented or those who are prisoners. Thus, legislation has been enacted to safeguard these people from being subject to forceful participation in research.

Another issue is whether someone found mentally ill can be executed for a crime in states that have the death penalty. Some state courts have ruled that criminals could not be forcibly medicated in order to make them competent for involuntary execution.

99. Can genetic information be abused?

In Part 4 on genetics, some of the eugenic movement was described. Psychiatrists were prominent in using superficial genetic statistics to suggest that sterilizing and then exterminating people who had "inherited" mental illness would be best for society. We need to proceed cautiously given the historical potential for use of genetic information to scapegoat religious, minority ethnic, and other groups. Many possibilities for abuse of genetic information are looming in the future, since with advanced technology, we can now determine the variants of genes that are present in embryos. What harm will we be doing in the future if certain variants are not allowed to continue according to the rules of evolution and natural selection?

The movie *Gattaca* was provocative and went relatively unnoticed. It was a startling look at what could happen in the future, depicting a "genetically enhanced" population of people who discriminated against those who were born by natural unions of men and women. This scenario may be more of a reality, given today's technology, than simply science fiction. Other abuses have to do with the public use of genetic information if it is known at birth. Could health insurance companies and life insurance salespersons refuse to insure individuals who have inherited the probability of getting certain diseases? Will there be job discrimination, education discrimination, and so on? Instead of the current cultural, ethnic, and racial discrimination, a new form of "genetic" discrimination could occur. These are all things to be prepared for and to govern against by legislation.

100. What support groups, books, and Web sites can I go to for help?

A list of support groups, Web sites, and books can be found under Resources. This book has been about public awareness of schizophrenia and is written so that the abuses based only on scientific half-truths will not occur. Schizophrenia is on the extreme edge of the wide range of what the world calls "normality." However it has been observed in each culture and at each point in time. It is an illness by virtue of the pain and destruction it causes to those afflicted. With the eventual development of future medications that target its biology, there is hope that this illness can be prevented. No one should feel shame or be stigmatized because he or she suffers from schizophrenia; rather patients should receive the best treatment from those who are trained to give it and then live their lives to their best potential.

Support Groups

The most prominent support group in the United States is the National Alliance on Mental Illness (NAMI), which has local chapters throughout the United States. The national office is located at:

Colonial Place Three
2107 Wilson Boulevard, Suite 300
Arlington, VA 22201-3042
Phone: 1-703-524-7600
Information helpline: 1-800-950-6264
Web site: www.NAMI.org

In the United Kingdom, the largest support group is Schizophrenia, a National Emergency (SANE), which is located at:

1st Floor Cityside House
40 Adler Street
London, E1 1EE
Phone: 020-7375-1002
E-mail: info@sane.org.uk
Web site: www.sane.org.uk

For emergency help, they provide a phone line called SANEline in the United Kingdom (0845-767-8000), which is also available by e-mail (sanemail@sane.org.uk).

In Canada, a useful source for support is the Schizophrenia Society of Canada, located at:

100-4 Fort Street
Winnapeg, MB R3C1C4, Canada
Phone: 204-786-1616
Fax: 204-783-4898
E-mail: info@schizophrenia.ca
Web site: www.schizophrenia.ca

Similar organizations exist in other countries as well.

Support internationally can be found through the World Fellowship for Schizophrenia and Allied Disorders, located at:

19 MacPherson Avenue
Toronto, Ontario, M5R 1W7, Canada
Phone: 1-416-961-2855
E-mail: info@world-schizophrenia.org
Web site: www.world-schizophrenia.org

Recommended Books

The following books that provide further information about schizophrenia and related disorders can provide comfort for families, friends, and individuals who have been diagnosed with schizophrenia.

Andreasen NC (2001). *Brave New Brain: Conquering Mental Illness in the Era of the Genome*. Oxford: Oxford University Press.

Jamison KR (2009). *Nothing Was the Same: A Memoir*. New York: Alfred A. Knopf.

Jamison KR (1995). *An Unquiet Mind: A Memoir of Mood and Madness*. New York: Alfred A. Knopf.

Jamison KR (1999). *Night Falls Fast: Understanding Suicide*. New York: Alfred A. Knopf.

Saks ER (2007). *The Center Cannot Hold: My Journey Through Madness*. New York: Harper and Row Publishers, Inc.

Torrey EF (2006). *Surviving Schizophrenia: A Manual for Families, Consumers, and Providers*, 5th ed. New York: Quill, Harper Collins.

Torrey EF (1998). *Out of the Shadows: Confronting America's Mental Illness Crisis*, 2nd ed. New York: John Wiley & Sons.

Recommended Web Sites

National Institute of Mental Health: www.nimh.nih.gov

National Alliance for Research on Schizophrenia and Depression (NARSAD): www.NARSAD.org

The Schizophrenia Research Forum: www.schizophreniaforum.org

The Schizophrenia International Research Society: www.schizophreniaresearchsociety.org

BIBLIOGRAPHY

American Psychiatric Association (2000). *Diagnostic and Statistical Manual of Mental Disorders*, 4th ed., text revision (DSM-IV-TR). Washington, DC: American Psychiatric Association Press.

Andreasen NC (2001). *Brave New Brain: Conquering Mental Illness in the Era of the Genome*. Oxford: Oxford University Press.

Aschaffenburg G (ed.). (1911–1928). Dementia praecox oder die Gruppe der Schizofrenien. *Handbuch der Psychiatrie*. Leipzig and Vienna.

Bak M, Myin-Germeys I, Hanssen M, et al. (2003). When does experience of psychosis result in a need for care? A prospective general population study. *Schizophr Bull* 29(2):349–358.

Chopra D (1991). *Unconditional Life: Discovering the Power to Fulfill Your Dreams*. New York: Bantam Books.

Crow TJ (1990). The continuum of psychosis and its genetic origins. *Br J Psychiatry* 156:788–797.

Crow TJ (1997). Is schizophrenia the price that Homo sapiens pays for language? *Schizophr Res* 28:127–141.

Crow TJ (2000). Schizophrenia as the price that Homo sapiens pays for language: a resolution of the central paradox in the origin of the species. *Brain Res Brain Res Rev* 31:118–129.

Crow TJ, Done DJ. (1986). Age of onset of schizophrenia in siblings: a test of the contagion hypothesis. *Psychiatry Res*. 18(2):107–117.

DeLisi LE (ed.) (1990). *Depression in Schizophrenia*. Washington, DC: American Psychiatric Association Press.

DeLisi LE (2000). Unifying the concept of psychosis through brain morphology. In: Maneros A, Angst J (eds.). (2000). *Bipolar Disorders: 100 Years After Manic Depressive Insanity*. The Netherlands: Kluwer.

DeLisi LE (2001). Speech disorder in schizophrenia: review of the literature and new study of the relation to uniquely human capacity for language. *Schizophr Bull* 27:481–496.

DeLisi LE (2008). The effect of cannabis on the brain: can it cause brain anomalies that lead to increased risk for schizophrenia? *Curr Opin Psychiatry* 21(2):140–150.

DeLisi LE (2008). The concept of progressive change in schizophrenia: implications for understanding schizophrenia. *Schizophrenia Bulletin* 34(2):312–321.

DeLisi LE, Crow TJ (1989). Evidence for an X chromosome locus for schizophrenia. *Schizophr Bull* 15:431–440.

El-Hai J (2004). *The Lobotomist: A Maverick Medical Genius and His Tragic Quest to Rid the World of Mental Illness.* Hoboken, NJ: John Wiley & Sons.

Faulks S (2005). *Human Traces.* London: Hutchinson, The Random House Group, Ltd.

Fink M (1999). *Electroshock: Healing Mental Illness.* Oxford: Oxford University Press.

Geller JL, Harris M (1994). *Women of the Asylum.* New York: Doubleday Anchor Books.

Gottesman II (1991). *Schizophrenia Genesis: The Origins of Madness.* New York: WH Freeman.

Gottesman II, Shields J (1982). *Schizophrenia: The Epigenetic Puzzle.* Cambridge: Cambridge University Press.

Gould SJ (1981). *The Mismeasure of Man.* New York: W.W. Norton and Company.

Henig RM (2000). *The Monk in the Garden.* New York: Houghton Mifflin.

Hoffman RE, Hawkins KA, Gueorguieva R, et al. (2003). Transcranial magnetic stimulation of left temporoparietal cortex and medication-resistant auditory hallucinations. *Arch Gen Psychiatry* 60:49–56.

Isaac RJ, Armat VC (1990, 2000). *Madness in the Streets: How Psychiatry and the Law Abandoned the Mentally Ill.* Treatment Advocacy Center. Free Press.

Jamison KR (1995). *An Unquiet Mind: A Memoir of Mood and Madness.* New York: Alfred A. Knopf.

Jamison KR (1999). *Night Falls Fast: Understanding Suicide.* New York: Alfred A. Knopf.

Johnstone EC, Crow TJ, Frith DC, Husband J, Krel L (1976). Cerebral ventricular size and cognitive impairment in schizophrenia. *Lancet* 2:924–926.

Kasanetz EF (1979). Tecnica per investigare il ruolo di fattori ambientale sulla genesi della schizophrenia. *Riv Psicol Anal* 10:193–202.

Kety SS, Rosenthal D, Wender PH, Schulsinger F (1968). The types and prevalences of mental illness in the biological and adoptive families of adopted schizophrenics. In: Rosenthal D, Kety SS (eds.). *The Transmission of Schizophrenia.* Oxford: Pergammon, 345–362.

Kingdon DG, Turkington D (1995). *Cognitive Behavioral Therapy for Schizophrenia*, new ed. Psychology Press.

Kraepelin E (1899). *Etiology of Dementia Praecox, Lehrbuch Der Psychitarie*, 6th ed. Barth, Lepzig.

Kraepelin E (1907). *Etiology of Dementia Praecox, Lehrbuch Der Psychitarie*, 7th ed. Livingstone, Edinburgh.

Kraepelin E (1919). In: *Dementia Praecox and Paraphrenia.* Barclay RM, translator. New York, NY: Krieger.

Menninger KA (1926). Influenza and schizophrenia: an analysis of post-influenzal "dementia praecox" as of 1918 and five years later. *Am J Psychiatry* 5:469–529.

Nasar S (1998). *A Beautiful Mind.* New York: Simon and Schuster.

Nasrallah HA, Smeltzer DJ (2003). *Contemporary Diagnosis and Management of the Patient with Schizophrenia.* Handbooks in Healthcare Company.

Reeder C, Wykes T (2005). *Cognitive Remediation Therapy for Schizophrenia.* London: Routledge.

Rosenthal D (ed.) (1963). *The Genain Quadruplets: A Case Study and Theoretical Analysis of Heredity and Environment in Schizophrenia.* New York: Basic Books.

Rosenthal D, Wender PH, Kety SS, Welner J, Schulsinger F (1968). Schizophrenic's offspring reared in adoptive homes. In: Rosenthal D, Kety SS (eds.). *The Transmission of Schizophrenia.* Oxford: Pergammon, 377–391.

Torrey EF (1980). *Schizophrenia and Civilization.* New York: Aronson.

Torrey EF (1984). *The Roots of Treason: Ezra Pound and the Secret of St. Elizabeth's.* New York: McGraw-Hill Book Company.

Torrey EF (1988). *Nowhere to Go: The Tragic Odyssey of the Homeless Mentally Ill.* New York: Harper & Row.

Torrey EF (1998). *Out of the Shadows: Confronting America's Mental Illness Crisis*, 2nd ed. New York: John Wiley & Sons.

Torrey EF (2001). *Surviving Schizophrenia: A Manual for Families, Consumers, and Providers*, 4th ed. New York: Quill.

Torrey EF, Miller J (2001). *The Invisible Plague: The Rise of Mental Illness from 1750 to the Present.* New Brunswick, NJ: Rutgers University Press.

Torrey EF, Peterson MR (1976). The viral hypothesis of schizophrenia. *Schizophr Bull* 2:136–146.

Verdoux H, van Os J (2002). Psychotic symptoms in non-clinical populations and the continuum of psychosis. *Schizophr Res* 54:59–65.

Whitaker R (2002). *Mad In America: Bad Science, Bad Medicine, and The Enduring Mistreatment of the Mentally Ill.* Perseus Publishing Co.

Glossary

Alzheimer's disease: One of a few progressive brain diseases that has been more frequently diagnosed recently in older people who appear disoriented, have memory loss for recent things, and have difficulty communicating properly with others. It consists of specific characteristic changes in the brain that can be seen only by autopsy after death, but MRI scans can also be revealing. The usual signs that will appear are large ventricles and atrophy of a region of the brain crucial for remembering, the hippocampus. Other parts of the brain can also be affected. Thus, a person with Alzheimer's disease has trouble remembering what happened one minute ago and has difficulty forming sentences and speaking, eventually progressing to the inability to take care of his or her basic needs.

Antipsychotic: Any medication that specifically suppresses the positive symptoms of hallucinations and delusions. This medication can also be useful in other conditions as a strong tranquilizer.

Atypical antipsychotic medications: These are newer medications that were put on the market by the drug companies beginning in the 1990s for use in schizophrenia and schizoaffective disorder. They are commonly called "the second generation" drugs. Because they have different biochemical effects in the brain compared to the older drugs, such as Thorazine or Haldol, and thus are less likely to cause the typical motor disturbances seen with these drugs, they have been called "atypical."

Bipolar affective disorder: A psychiatric condition characterized by mood swings that occur episodically. Sometimes, particularly when very "high" (manic), people with bipolar disorder can have many of the characteristic positive symptoms of schizophrenia.

Catatonia: A condition that is characterized by extremes in behavior, of which the individual appears to be unaware. These behaviors include being mute or in a stupor and immobile, or, at the other extreme, being in an excitatory state of an extreme frenzy or agitation. This condition is not specific to schizophrenia; however, when it is periodically present in someone who has other characteristics of schizophrenia, it is then diagnosed as the subtype called "catatonic schizophrenia."

Chromosome: A structure present in the nucleus of every cell of the body of any living thing and containing genes. It is shaped like a long cylinder separated into two arms that are held together in the approximate middle by a structure called the centromere. The two arms have been named "p" and "q", and the length of the cylinder has been quantified by the distance from the distal tip of the "p" arm. The "p" arm is usually the shorter of the two chromosome arms. The total distance of one chromosome is measured in centimorgans (cM), named after the scientist who worked out the method for measuring it, Morgan. In addition, people who view chromosomes under the microscope have noticed differences in the dark and light constitutions of the chromosome that may mean breaks in where clusters of genes start and end. Thus, a method was developed for counting these bands. The band numbers begin from the centromere and go distally, using consecutively higher numbers on each arm. These two methods of measuring chromosomes and their size then give geneticists the ability to know where different genes are located on the chromosome. Thus, when a gene is located on chromosome 6q21, 150 cM from pter, this means it is on the sixth chromosome on the larger arm (the "q" arm) and within the 21st band down on that arm. Its exact distance from the distal tip of the "p" arm is 150 centimorgans. More and more information given to the public will now be in these terms; for example: "A gene for XX disease has been found by researchers on chromosome 6q21."

Cognition: The quality of the mind that allows animals to think, reason, and manipulate their environment to survive. Cognition can be measured by psychological tests. Of course, the tests are much simpler for nonhuman animals and are most complicated for humans. The well-known IQ (intelligence quotient) is one measure of human cognition.

Cognitive behavioral therapy (CBT): A brief form of treatment based on the principle that the way one thinks about something causes actions. Thus, it is focused on changing thinking patterns that lead to disruptive behavior. Several different techniques are available for this. This form of therapy is used for a variety of psychiatric disorders. Unlike the way it sounds, this is not a type of therapy that trains people to improve their cognition or intellectual abilities.

Command hallucinations: Imaginary voices that tell the hearer what to do.

Computed tomography (CT): A form of X-ray that is able to view the brain in more detail than a standard skull X-ray. However, it has been largely replaced by MRI as a diagnostic tool to examine details of the brain.

The advantage CT has over MRI is that it detects bone change, whereas MRI views the brain tissue, and is not sensitive to bone. CT scans may be preferable to MRI scans when patients have metal implants in their bodies or cardiac pacemakers, as the magnets used for MRI may dislodge these devices. CT does not use magnets, but rather radiation.

Copy number variation (CNV): A CNV is a segment of DNA in which a difference in the number of copies of sequences has been found by comparing DNA from two or more people. These may be inherited or caused by de novo mutations. CNVs are common throughout each person's genome. Sometimes if they occur within genes, they may change their function and could be pathologic.

Cortex (cerebral cortex): The outer portion of the brain. It consists mostly of the "gray matter" that contains nerve cells.

Delusion: A false belief based on faulty judgment about one's environment.

Depression: A major psychiatric condition characterized by profound sadness all day. It is usually accompanied by physical symptoms, such as loss of appetite, loss of sleep, and slowness in movements and speech. If the condition continues as long as 2 weeks without relief and interferes with a person's ability to function, it is then called major depression.

Disorganization syndrome: A set of symptoms related to general disorganization (i.e., speech that is mixed-up or not getting to the point and behavioral disorganization). These symptoms are now considered a separate cluster.

Deoxyribonucleic acid (DNA): Inherited material made of different nucleic acids put together in the form of a triple helix. It consists of a long polymer with a deoxyribose and phosphate backbone and four different bases: adenine, guanine, cytosine, and thymine. Genes are made up of DNA and the variation in genes between individuals depends on the sequence of these nucleic acids in an individual's genes. Chromosomes are made up of sequences of DNA with genes intermittently spaced along the chromosome and separated by segments of DNA that do not represent an inherited function (or genes). DNA makes up the chromosomes of all animals and plants and many viruses.

Dopamine: One of the chemical substances that is important for conveying "messages" between nerve cells in the brain.

DSM-IV: *Diagnostic and Statistical Manual of Mental Disorders*, developed by leading clinical psychiatrists in the United States for systematically evaluating psychiatric patients and assigning diagnoses to groups of symptoms. There have been four major separate revisions of this code of diagnoses since its inception and currently psychiatrists are working on the *DSM-V*. The current *DSM-IV* has five axes: Axis I is for major diagnoses, Axis II is for personality disorders,

Axis III is for medical conditions, Axis IV is for level of stressors, and Axis V is a measure of general global functioning.

Dyskinesia: Difficulty in performing movements voluntarily.

Electroconvulsive therapy: A type of treatment that gives a series of electrical shocks to regions of the brain. Treatment is given in sessions that are separated by several days. The way it exerts its effects is unknown. However, it is not dangerous or painful and is accompanied by an anesthesia when administered. The only known side effect is memory loss subsequent to the treatment. It is mainly used for depression, but can produce temporary improvement in people who have schizophrenia, particularly with persistent painful thoughts and hallucinations that don't disappear with medication.

Electroencephalogram (EEG): A type of test whereby electrodes are placed on several areas of the head and recordings are made of the brain's electrical activity.

Endophenotype: ***See Intermediate phenotype***

Enzymes: Proteins in the body that digest other substances through biochemical reactions. They are the "tools" of metabolism.

Estrogen: A female hormone that is produced in the female organs (ovaries). It is produced in different amounts throughout the menstrual cycle and is reduced after menopause.

Family therapy: A type of treatment that focuses on alleviating problems the entire family entity has interacting with each other. Family therapy used to be popular in the 1960s and 1970s to treat schizophrenia. This therapy was based on the premise that the patient was the "family" and not any one individual within in it. Thus no one person was labeled as "ill," but pathologic family interactions were thought to be the cause of one person becoming ill and thus those interactions needed treatment. This is no longer thought to be an acceptable treatment for schizophrenia. However, support for families having a member with schizophrenia can be helpful so that members are better able to deal with his/her illness.

Fecundity: Bearing children.

Fertility: Having the normal biology that gives one the ability to bear children.

Fish oil: Omega-3 fatty acids. These substances are important for the building of the lining of nerves. For good functioning of the nervous system, it is important that these fatty acids are in abundance. Fish oil is a commercial product that can be bought in health food stores at various levels of purity and has been advertised as a "cure-all" for many conditions; most claims have not been substantiated scientifically.

Functional MRI (fMRI): A brain scan that shows actions taking place in the brain in response to a stimulus. The stimulus could be anything, such as voluntary movement of the fingers or thinking about or distinguishing the meaning of a set of words.

Gene: A functional unit of heredity that is in a fixed place in the structure of a chromosome.

Geneticists: Scientists who study the inheritance of traits in humans, animals, or plants.

Glutamine/glutamate: An amino acid that is a building block of proteins. It is also by itself one of the major neurotransmitters in the brain (i.e., transmits information from cell to cell); by stimulating the activity of the cells, it excites them into activity.

Gray matter: The brownish-gray nerve tissue of the brain and spinal cord that contains the nerve cells.

Hallucination: The experience of something from any of the five senses that is not occurring in reality (e.g., hearing voices when no one is there speaking, seeing images of things that are not really there, smelling something that is not there, feeling something touch one's body when that thing is not actually there, or tasting something that one is not eating).

Hippocampus: A relatively small brain structure that lies deep within the temporal lobe and is thought to be crucial for memory. It has been given this name because of its unusual curved shape.

Homo sapiens: The scientific designation for modern human beings.

Immunoglobulins: The proteins that help the body respond to foreign substances and infections.

Insanity: Mental malfunctioning or unsoundness of mind that produces lack of judgment to the degree that the individual cannot manage his or her affairs or conform to social standards. This term is also used in criminal law, to suggest mental conditions or defects that may relieve a person from the legal consequences of his or her acts that break laws. People may then be found not guilty by reason of insanity, which implies that they do not know the difference between what is right and what is wrong.

Intermediate phenotype: Sometimes also called an "endophenotype." It is the trait in genetic terms that a gene is responsible for more directly producing something else that then leads to the clinical illness itself. This trait then leads to the development of the clinical illness or makes a person more vulnerable to getting the illness. For example, an intermediate phenotype for schizophrenia may be a change in the structure of the brain that in turn may put someone at risk for getting schizophrenia. An intermediate phenotype is considered to be something that is closer to (more directly a consequence of) the actual gene than the symptoms of the disease itself.

Linkage: A genetic term that signifies a relationship between two or more genes on the same chromosome that are relatively close together so that sometimes the variations in the traits that each represents are inherited together in the same individual. When genes are linked in a genetic sense, they are close together on a chromosome and thus the inherited variations in them are more likely than chance to occur together in the same individual.

Lobotomy: The surgical division of one or more brain tracts. It is usually referred to as cutting nerves that run from the frontal lobe to the thalamus in the brain. It has been done in various ways, most often by inserting a needle above the nose in between the eyes. It is also known as leukotomy.

Magnetic resonance imaging (MRI): A method to examine the tissue of the brain using a magnetic field and computer system. The machine itself consists of a horizontal tube powered by a giant magnet. The patient having an MRI scan lies on his or her back and slides into the tube on a special table. Once inside, the patient is scanned.

Magnetic resonance spectroscopy (MRS): A type of MRI scan that examines chemical spectras in the brain. The chemicals examined are those present in the structure of membranes or metabolic activity in nerve cells and between cells.

Manic behavior: Excitatory behavior with a rapid pace in both speech and movements. This behavior is sometimes accompanied by grandiose delusions and feelings of such well being that the individual thinks he/she has special abilities and powers. Mania is also frequently accompanied by little need for sleep and behaviors that are reckless and tend to produce harm to the person having such behavior.

Microarray: An orderly arrangement of DNA samples to identify many genes at one time. They can contain thousands of genes on one small plate or "chip." An experiment with a single DNA chip or microarray can provide researchers information on thousands of genes simultaneously. There are also RNA arrays that can provide information about gene expression.

Monozygotic twins: Twins born at the same time who originate from the splitting of the same egg after it has been fertilized. The DNA is identical in both twins; and thus the twins are sometimes referred to as identical.

Negative symptoms: Those characteristics of psychiatric illness that present as withdrawn behavior, an expressionless face, a lack of initiative, a lack of interest, slow speech (and not saying much when talking), slowed thoughts, and slowed movements. Sometimes these symptoms are confused with either depression or side effects of medication.

Neurodevelopmental: Happening during the growth and formation of different structures of the brain. This may be prenatally, during childhood, or even through adolescence and early adulthood.

Neuroleptic: Any medication that will cause catalepsy when given to animals. This name is used to label all drugs that have an effect on reducing the symptoms of schizophrenia. They are sometimes known as the "major tranquilizers."

Neuroleptic malignant syndrome (NMS): A severe, although rare, side effect of neuroleptic treatment; its cause is unknown. It begins with rigidity or worsening in psychiatric symptoms despite increases in medication. Some of the warning signs are fast heart beat, high fluctuating blood pressure, tremors, sweating, and fever. Cessation of neuroleptic therapy is the only treatment. It is a serious medical emergency that requires immediate treatment.

Paranoia: The feeling that other people are doing harmful things to oneself or thinking about doing such, or that others are watching or observing oneself unnecessarily. This is a general mistrust of other people for no sensible reason that can develop into extreme delusions.

Pharmacotherapy: Treatment of disease through the use of drugs.

Phenotype: The trait that is expressed by a gene. For example, having blue eyes or brown eyes would be phenotypes. The clinical disorder called schizophrenia may also be a "phenotype" in genetic studies.

Pneumoencephalography: An X-ray picture of the brain taken by injection of air into the cerebral ventricular space. Prior to the advent of CT and MRI scanning, this method was used to detect whether a patient had brain atrophy. This method is no longer in use.

Positive symptoms: Considered the active symptoms of hallucinations and delusions of schizophrenia.

Positron emission tomography (PET) scan: A radiologic procedure that measures the metabolism of a radiolabeled substance. A substance, which is known to enter the brain relatively rapidly, is radiolabeled and then injected into a subject's bloodstream. Pictures are then taken of the brain with the regions metabolizing the injected substance "lighting up." PET scans are valuable tools to detect early brain tumors and have been useful in Alzheimer's research. However, they are difficult and expensive to perform, requiring a cyclotron to manufacture the radiolabeled compound, and they are also uncomfortable for patients. Thus, they have not been popular in recent years among schizophrenia researchers.

Premorbid: The time period before any symptoms of a disorder, including subtle signs, have developed.

Prenatal: The period between conception and birth.

Prodrome: An early or premonitory symptom of a disease. If true specific prodromal symptoms are known, one can detect the illness early. These symptoms signify that the disease will be almost certain.

Psychotherapy: Therapy that is performed by talking to the patient in various ways, either by helping the patient have insight into his/her actions or by providing support and encouragement to deal with life's problems. This may be used in combination with pharmaco- or other types of therapies. Psychotherapy is not considered a substitute for good pharmacotherapy for schizophrenia.

Psychotic: A condition defined by losing touch with reality or having delusions (i.e., false beliefs) and hallucinations. Psychotic individuals often exhibit bizarre and risky behavior and do not seem to be aware that they are doing anything unusual.

Residual: Having some nonspecific symptoms (usually negative symptoms) but no longer active psychotic ones.

Ribonucleic acid (RNA): A nucleic acid polymer that plays an important role in the process that translates genetic information from deoxyribonucleic acid (DNA) into protein products. It is found in both the nucleus and cytoplasm of cells. RNA is a polymer with a ribose and phosphate backbone and four different bases: adenine, guanine, cytosine, and uracil. There are different types of RNA: mRNA (messenger RNA: carries a DNA message into the cytoplasm from the nucleus); tRNA (transfer RNA: carries amino acids to the mRNA and ribosomes); rRNA (ribosomal RNA: responsible for protein synthesis in the ribosomes that are in the cytoplasm of the cell).

Schizoaffective: Having prominent symptoms both of schizophrenia and of depression and/or mania. However, they do not always completely coincide; rather, they tend to overlap in episodes. Sometimes when someone is diagnosed with schizoaffective disorder, it is difficult for psychiatrists to decide whether they predominantly have schizophrenia or they predominantly have bipolar disorder. Thus, this disorder lies somewhere in between both disorders on a continuum of symptoms. Researchers do not know whether this disorder has unique biology or is related to schizophrenia, bipolar disorder, or both.

Schizophrenia: A psychotic disorder usually characterized by withdrawal from reality and social interactions, illogical and disorganized patterns of thinking and speaking, multiple delusions, and hallucinations, and accompanied in varying degrees by other emotional, behavioral, or intellectual disturbances of the brain. Schizophrenia is associated with dopamine and other neurochemical imbalances in the brain and structural and functional defects of the frontal and temporal lobes. It is thought to be caused by genetic and other biological factors.

Schizophreniform: Having the symptoms of schizophrenia, but too early in the course of illness to tell whether the symptoms are of a schizophrenia illness.

Segmental duplications: Repeats of segments of DNA sequences along a chromosome.

Serotonin: A hormone found in the brain, platelets, digestive tract, and pineal gland. It acts both as a neurotransmitter (a substance that nerves use to send messages to one another) and a vasoconstrictor (a substance that causes blood vessels to narrow). A reduction of serotonin in the brain is thought to be a cause of depression.

Stigma: Literally a "mark"; something visible to others that sets an individual apart from others whether for justified or unjustified reasons.

Superior temporal gyrus: A portion of the temporal lobe of the brain that has many functions related to language, including hearing it and speaking it.

Tranquilizer: Any drug that is used to calm or pacify an anxious and/or agitated person. There are minor and major classes of tranquilizers that have different chemical properties and are indicated for different psychiatric conditions. The minor ones are for anxiety in a person who has not lost a sense of reality but who needs calming. Major tranquilizers are the class of drugs used for psychotic symptoms.

Ventricles: As this term applies to the brain, the spaces connecting throughout the brain that provide a system for the circulation of the fluid present in the brain called cerebrospinal fluid. The ventricles in the brain consist of the lateral, third, and fourth ventricles; they connect to the spinal column and bathe the spinal cord.

White matter: The whitish brain and spinal cord tissue composed mostly of nerve fibers and its shiny protective coat called myelin.

Working memory: A contemporary term for short-term memory. It is thought of as an active system for temporarily storing and manipulating information needed for conducting complex tasks such as learning, reasoning, and comprehending things. There are two components of working memory: storage and central executive functions. The two storage systems within working memory are for temporary storage of verbal and visual information. The central executive function is thought to be a process that is very active and responsible for the selection, initiation, and termination of processing for the storing and retrieving of memories.

Index

C

D

E

F

G

H

Q

R

S